The Myofascial Release Manual

Second Edition

The Myofascial Release Manual

Second Edition

Carol J. Manheim, MS, MEd, PT
Plantation Plaza Therapy Center
12-C Carriage Lane
Charleston, SC

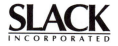

SLACK
INCORPORATED

Note to the Reader

Although I would prefer to write in a gender neutral language, I was unable to do so. I regret that there are no concise or appropriate gender neutral terms that could have been used. For clarity and ease of reading, the male gender pronouns have been used to refer to my model. The female gender pronoun was used whenever it was more appropriate to my experience.

Managing Editor: Amy E. Drummond
Publisher: John H. Bond
Project Editor: Debra L. Clarke

The procedures and practices described in this book should be implemented in a manner consistent with the professional standards set for the circumstances that apply in each specific situation. Every effort has been made to confirm the accuracy of information presented and to correctly relate generally accepted practices.

The authors, editor, and publisher cannot accept responsibility for errors or exclusions or for the outcome of the application of the material herein. There is no expressed or implied warranty of this book or information imparted by it.

The work SLACK publishes is peer reviewed. Prior to publication, recognized leaders in the field, educators, and clinicians provide important feedback on the concepts and content that we publish. We welcome feedback on this work.

Manheim, Carol J.
    The myofascial release manual/Carol J. Manheim.
  2nd ed.
      p. cm.
  Includes bibliographic references and index.
  ISBN 1-55642-241-5 wire-o
  ISBN 1-55642-249-0 perfect bound
  1. Manipulation (Therapeutics) 2. Stretch (Physiology) 3. Physical Therapy
  I. Title
[DNLM 1. Physical Therapy--methods. 2. Fascia--physiology 3. Manipulation, Orthopedic--methods.
4. Muscles--physiology. 5. Relaxation Techniques. WB 460 M2777m 1994]
    RM724.M34 1994
615.8'2--dc20   94-13677
                                                                      CIP

Printed in the United States of America

Published by: SLACK Incorporated
              6900 Grove Road
              Thorofare, NJ 08086-9447 USA
              Telephone: 856-848-1000
              Fax: 856-853-5991
              World Wide Web: http://www.slackinc.com

Last digit is print number: 10 9 8 7 6 5 4

Dedication

To

my patients who allow me to learn, practice and refine my skills of Myofascial Release

my students who make me put into words the sensations and techniques of Myofascial Release

my children

Contents

Acknowledgments

Portions of this book previously appeared in *Myofascial Release: A Nontraditional Approach To Stretching*, published by Forum Medicum in the Postgraduate Advances in Physical Therapy Continuing Education Course II, under the sponsorship of the American Physical Therapy Association.

Diane K. Lavett, PhD was my co-author for the first edition of *The Myofascial Release Manual*. Without her vision and organization, this book would never have come into being.

Patti Bagg, PT and Annie Ruth Wright assisted with the preparation of the first edition and the photography for it. Ron, Paul and Julie Kaplan assisted in the next two photography sessions and were the early manuscript reviewers. Lisa Razmyar, PTA has provided invaluable assistance in the preparation of this second edition.

Michael Whittemore, photographer, has been an extremely important participant in the dynamic process of bringing clarity and movement to the still photographs of this technique. Through his artistic vision, he has been able to demonstrate muscle structure being stretched in minute detail.

About the Author

Carol J. Manheim received her MS degree from Case Western Reserve University and her MEd in clinical counseling from The Citadel.

She is the co-author of *The Myofascial Release Manual, First Edition* and *Craniosacral Therapy and Somato-Emotional Release: The Self-Healing Body*.

Ms. Manheim has presented papers on Myofascial Release and the psychological effects of manual therapies at the World Confederation of Physical Therapy and at the national convention of the American Physical Therapy Association. In addition, she has presented lectures on body memory and physically facilitated abreactions.

She is a member of the American Physical Therapy Association, the Neurodevelopmental Treatment Association and is certified in the Treatment of Adults with Hemiplegia. She is also a member of The International Society for Behavioral Science in Physical Therapy, The International Society for the Study of Multiple Personality and Dissociative Disorders, the American Association for Counseling and Development, the American Mental Health Counselors Association, and Chi Iota Sigma, a national counseling honorary society.

Ms. Manheim is currently in private practice in Charleston, South Carolina.

Introduction

by Sam Kegerreis, MS, PT, ATC

Myofascial therapy can be defined as "the facilitation of mechanical, neural, and psychophysiological adaptive potential as interfaced via the myofascial system."[1] This inclusive definition attempts to acknowledge the wide variety of techniques currently taught under the myofascial signature. Myofascial procedures vary significantly, ranging from prolonged stretching and soft tissue mobilization to subtle indirect techniques. Such ambiguity is obviously frustrating to the uninitiated clinician as well as to the researcher attempting to quantify suggested benefits.

It must be understood that myofascial therapy represents a philosophy of care rather than a series of techniques. Characteristics common to most myofascial work include manual contact from clinician to client and an attempt to link the input of the therapist to the inherent corrective capacity of the patient. Myofascial therapy is ideally *not* something one does *to* a client. Most experienced manual therapists readily acknowledge that treatment procedures are inseparable from evaluation. Patient response is constantly monitored and used as an indicator to guide further care. A hallmark of most myofascial work is the attempt to entrain the patient and clinician in such a way as to permit the patient's response to manual contact to facilitate the treatment. This approach requires the clinician to relinquish specific intent and to rely on intuition seldom valued in present allopathic spheres. Perceived benefits are grounded in the concept of inherent neural and mechanical plasticity as enhanced by a product of interaction between clinician and patient.

The exasperation of modern scientists when contemplating this phenomena is readily appreciated. How does one investigate cause and effect when neither intervention nor outcome can be finitely anticipated? Does a change occur in the patient's condition, and if so, can it be measured and maintained? If human contact facilitates an inherent tendency for desirable patient correction, exactly what role does the clinician play in directing this outcome? What unique qualities and experiences brought to the treatment process by the clinician or patient determine a desirable or undesirable response? Could it be that patient response is entirely placebo in nature, with respect to a touch-deprived society? And if so, do patients respond similarly to other forms of manual care?

Despite these and other concerns, myofascial therapy seems unusually resistant to the inevitable slow death traditionally reserved for fads that periodically infest the clinical arena. Myofascial therapy appears to be growing in popularity and in medical acceptance. It has been, at times, amusing to observe the frustration of accomplished clinicians as they find fault with their unresponsive, emotional, and seemingly mindless patients who claim to benefit from "myofascial nonsense" at the hands of less sophisticated practitioners.

When described in an inclusive manner, myofascial therapy is not a current fad so much as a dated concept that has recently been discovered by allopathic medicine via the vehicle of physical therapy. Osteopathic literature describing myofascial models appeared in the 1950's and was preceded by the contributions of Elisabeth Dicke (connective tissue massage) and Ida Rolf (structural integration). Lawrence Jones's strain and counterstrain, soft tissue mobilization, and many other contemporary schools of thought contain similar philosophies.[2,3] In addition, body workers of various experiential and educational backgrounds, ignored and unencumbered by scientific scrutiny, have utilized myofascial concepts for ages.[4]

The gap between myofascial consumers and myofascial critics will ideally one day be bridged by those with instincts common to both camps. However, a matter of much greater significance is the need to understand that the current controversy regarding myofascial therapy is but a microcosm of much larger debate involving competing perceptions as to the very nature of health and disease.

Biomedical and Infomedical Models

The basic differences between those on opposing sides of the myofascial issue are magnified by the inability to recognize an age-old controversy regarding the nature of health and disease. Western allopathic medicine, as described by Irby,[5] is based on a **biomedical model** influenced largely by Newtonian physics. Newtonian physics facilitates deductive reasoning and encourages specialization by advocating the breakdown of complex systems into smaller, more manageable units. Advances made utilizing this system have been considerable, perhaps at the expense of creating a naive perception of medical omnipotence. Accompanying this reductionistic perspective is an emphasis on pathology (versus the patient) and the Cartesian concept of mind/body dualism. Successes and failures are evaluated via biological outcomes such as ROM and strength, and little is left to mystery or chance. Another unfortunate side effect of this evolution is the tendency for patients to relinquish the responsibility for their health to medical deities rather than taking an active role in their own welfare.

A competing (and growing) model of health and disease can be traced to Hippocrates who urged his students to facilitate the natural healing capacity of each individual, rather than becoming enamored with the disease processes of the day.[6] This concept was embraced by perhaps the foremost physician of the 19th century, Sir William Osler, who pleaded that, "It is more important to know what sort of patient has a disease than what sort of disease a patient has."[7] C.S. Lewis[8] similarly wrote, "The magic is not in the medicine but in the patient's body—in the vis medicatrix nature, the recuperative or self-corrective energy of nature. What treatment does is to stimulate natural functions or to remove what hinders them." Irby[5] credits an advancing appreciation of quantum physics for the rebirth of this perspective. He states, "The reigning scientific model, derived from the first scientific revolution of Newtonian physics, produced biomedicine and experimental research design in education. The model emerging today is grounded in the second scientific revolution of Einstein's quantum physics and is creating **infomedicine** (acknowledgment of all phenomena: physical, biological, sociological, spiritual, and cultural) and ecological research in education."

Ingrained within the infomedical model is an appreciation of the interaction of multiple factors in the ultimate presentation of disease including mind/body relationships. Patients are valued for the inherent healing potential they uniquely possess, and they are held responsible for their own health, utilizing medical personnel as partners in this process. While biological outcomes remain important, they are meaningless unless directly related to functional change. A comparison of biomedical and infomedical models is shown here.

Biomedical Model	Infomedical Model
Newtonian Physics	Quantum Physics
Pathology Oriented	Patient (Process) Oriented
Reductionistic	Interdependency
Cartesian	Mind/Body Awareness
Clinician Responsibility	Patient Responsibility
Biological Outcomes	Functional Outcomes

Pathological Distinctions

Newtonian reasoning largely perceives pathology as a unidimensional threat to be analyzed and conquered. The dominant biomedical model functions well in dealing with **essentialistic** diagnoses. Examples of essentialistic diagnoses include fractures, bacterial infections, and joint dislocations. Each is clearly identified and, barring complications, can be expected to respond predictably to specific treatment regimes. However, by comparison, **nomanalistic** diagnoses tend to be multi-dimensional, less readily labeled, and more complex to treat. Examples of nomanalistic diagnoses include low back pain, reflex sympathetic dystrophy, and thoracic outlet syndrome. Irby[5] states, "There are diseases that afflict animals and humans that are predominantly biological in origin, and the biomedical model addresses these well. Second, there is another class of diseases that afflict humans alone and are predominantly biopsychocultural in origin. The infomedical model is best at investigating this class of disease."

Thus, the infomedical model embraces the complex interactions that constitute nomanalistic diagnosis and treatment. Traditional scientific inquiry is challenged to develop alternative methods of investigating this phenomena, and patients are encouraged to become partners in their own health care. Accountability is directly related to patient function.

The recent popularity of myofascial therapy is a logical consequence of the re-emergence of the infomedical health care model. It is within the context of the infomedical model that myofascial therapy should be most critically examined. Robert Ward, DO,[3] speaking of myofascial therapy adds, "Surprising help occurs in some situations with significant lack of success in seemingly similar cases. Many mysteries remain. Given these realities, the conclusion must be that disrupted neurohumoral, autonomic, and behavioral factors link soft tissue, arthrodial joints, and biomechanical changes in ambiguous ways." For reasons currently unknown, myofascial therapy appears to open a "pathway" for many patients suffering from recalcitrant nomanalistic complaints. Given the variety of techniques utilized it can be inferred that mechanical properties are but one of numerous mechanisms responsible for the empirical success of myofascial therapy. Much remains to be learned.

Structural Concepts

Fascia has been described as the most pervasive tissue in the body, representing a three-dimensional network from head to toe. Superficial fascia is a loosely knit, fibroelastic tissue attached to the undersurface of the skin. Vascular structures, adipose cells, and afferent receptors can be found in this layer, providing constant conscious and unconscious feedback to the central nervous system. Deep fascia varies in density, compartmentalizing the body and separating and surrounding visceral organs. Epimysium, perimysium, and endomysium represent fascial sheets contributing to efficiency in the development of muscle tension. Muscle represents between 70 and 85% of one's body weight, and perhaps more than any other organ, reflects and influences our ability to respond to the world around us. Muscle, with the help of its fascial binding, supplies the tension that gives life to our osseous framework. Muscle and fascia are functionally linked (myofascia), combining the properties of contractile and non-contractile tissue. Under load, fascia behaves mechanically with both plastic and elastic deformation, including the ability to change and lose energy when subjected to stress (hysteresis). Subserous fascia represents the deepest layer of fascia intimately surrounding and lubricating the internal viscera.

The function of the fascia has been largely underestimated. Fascia not only contributes contour to the body, but also provides lubrication between structures for movement (muscle play) and nutrition. Vessels and nerves are escorted throughout the body via fascial membranes contributing to metabolic homeostasis. Reflex mechanisms further contribute to neural function and development via receptors in subcutaneous fascia, the skin and connective tissues.

Tensegrity

The relationship of postural balance to efficient and pain-free musculoskeletal function has been admirably addressed by numerous authors.[9,10] Detrimental length-tension relationships have been associated with mechanical, neural, and psychological sources. Juhan[4] infers of adverse mechanical tension, "...the proper adjustment of length and tension in the connective tissues is a matter of extreme significance in the distribution of gravitational force throughout the body."

It is common to view upright skeletal posture in the manner that one visualizes the construction of a tall building, as a series of interlocking vertical and horizontal beams upon which the remaining structural material rests. Buckminster Fuller's concept of the geodesic dome takes issue with this model of vertical integrity pointing out the inefficiency of such structures. His **tensegrity** model consists of solid beams serving as spacers against tensional wires which actually become stronger in the presence of compressional force. One can easily appreciate which design is chosen by the body when observing the inability of a model skeleton to stand erect without extrinsic support. Without myofascial tension the human organism is incapable of upright posture. The body resists gravitational forces most efficiently when myofascial tension is balanced. Is there any wonder that the trapezius muscle reveals increased EMG activity at rest when attempting to restrain the forces imposed by forward head posture? The primary distinction between Fuller's model and that of human beings is that inorganic models do not think. Unless reacting to superimposed stresses, mechanical tension remains constant. The tensional qualities of **human tensegrity** units vary minute to minute (like blood pressure) in response to threats, real and imagined. The energy expended by individuals who admit "I just don't seem to know how to relax" is considerable. Unbalanced tension, its ultimate causes, and attempts to rectify the damage done by it are the stuff that the infomedical model is made of. Myofascial therapy is but one armament utilized by physical therapists in this battle.

Sam Kegerreis, MS, PT, ATC
Associate Professor of Physical Therapy
Krannert School of Physical Therapy
University of Indianapolis
Clinical Consultant
Methodist Sports Medicine Center
Indianapolis, IN

I

Fundamentals of Myofascial Release

Definition

Myofascial Release is a highly interactive stretching technique that requires feedback from the patient's body to determine the direction, force and duration of the stretch and to facilitate maximum relaxation of the tense tissues. Myofascial Release or myofascial stretching recognizes that a muscle cannot be isolated from the other structures of the body. All organs of the body are covered by fascia down to the individual myofibrils. Therefore, all "muscle stretching" is actually stretching of myofascial units. It is the philosophic base which separates Myofascial Release from other stretching techniques.

While using Myofascial Release techniques, the therapist monitors tissue tension by developing a kinesthetic link with the patient through touch. This link involves matching the inherent tissue movement, the rate and rhythm of the patient's respiration, the underlying neurophysiologic tissue tone and the more overt muscle tone. As the therapist becomes more adept at matching the patient's tone and tension, the therapist is able to detect subtle restrictions within individual myofascial units. As these areas are identified, gentle localized stretching is performed. In this manner, restrictions to efficient movement are located which cannot be either identified or eliminated using any other stretching technique. All malalignments which may predispose the patient to future injury are removed while treating the patient's current problem.

Thus, the therapist using Myofascial Release techniques works with the patient, not on the patient. The therapist is a facilitator, not an unquestionable expert. The therapist using Myofascial Release does not plan a treatment session in a step-by-step fashion, rather the therapist waits for guidance from the patient's body and follows the patient's lead. This philosophic stance takes the therapist out of the role of expert or god-figure and places the therapist on an even plane with the patient. It also allows the patient to participate as an equal in the treatment process. Thus, stretching of restricted tissues which impede efficient movement does not become a power play between the therapist and the patient. Instead, the philosophic orientation of myofascial stretching promotes patient cooperation and enlists the active participation of the patient in the healing process.

The goal of treatment using Myofascial Release is to facilitate the most efficient posture and movement patterns the patient can maintain. Postural and/or movement dysfunction is analyzed and treated in a holistic manner, recognizing that a limitation in one part of the body will have ramifications throughout the body. Progress is measured by improvement in postural symmetry, reduction in active myofascial trigger points, and increased fluidity of movement. Concrete range of motion measurements as well as postural photographs and verbal description of posture provide more objective documentation of progress.

Assumptions

To use the techniques described in this manual successfully, the therapist will have to make the following assumptions. First, the techniques of Myofascial Release work even though the exact mechanism is not yet known. Second, utilizing the feedback received from the patient's body, the therapist can effectively stretch restricted structures in a manner more comfortable to the patient than can be done with traditional stretching techniques, and without sacrificing the effectiveness of the stretch. Third, Myofascial Release removes restrictions that impede efficient movement. Fourth, as long as the therapist can feel restrictions through proprioceptive feedback from the patient's body, the actual structure of the restriction does not have to be known. Fifth, when there is a conflict between what you feel as feedback from the patient's body and what you see, what you feel is more accurate and more important. Sixth, when what the patient tells you is happening is different from what you are feeling, what you are feeling is more accurate. Remember that the patient's interpretation is prejudiced by what the patient may have been told or taught previously. Seventh, Myofascial Release is a very safe technique which prevents inadvertent over-stretching of the soft tissues of the body when the techniques are applied properly.

Soft tissue injuries, while widely diagnosed as strains, sprains or inflammation, receive minimal attention in the education of most physicians. Soft tissue injury is the injury which falls between the cracks of the medical specialties. For this reason, the patient with soft tissue injury may be seen by a general practitioner, an internist, an orthopedic surgeon, a neurologist, or a rheumatologist. Unfortunately for the patient, the medical treatment may mask or eliminate the pain while leaving the soft tissue restrictions or trigger points which can continue to cause inefficient posture and/or movement leading to resumption of the pain. Too often treatment is focused on the elimination of the symptom, which is pain, and not the origin of the pain. When both the pain and dysfunction are treated at the same time, the recurrence of the problem is less likely.[11]

How many times do our patients tell us we are the first to place our hands on the patient's body to palpate the soft tissues? How many times do we hear that we are the first to examine the patient's ability to move? How many times do we hear that we are the first to listen to the patient's story in an effort to assess the nature of the injury? How many times do we hear that we are the first to confirm that patients have, in fact, a physical problem and not a problem that is "all in their heads"?

As physical therapists, we must let our education and sensitive hands guide us in the treatment of our patients who are in pain. Our treatments need to be directed and mediated by the information we gain from our patients verbally and nonverbally, through touch. If we do not touch, do not sense through touch the pain of our patients, do not let the pain determine our treatment, then our patients will continue to suffer from pain and dysfunction, and they will be prevented from recovering as fully as possible from their injuries.

As physical therapists, we are uniquely qualified to address the problems of soft tissue injury and treatment. We have learned to see under the skin with our fingers. We have learned to detect dysfunction that other medical professionals cannot see because they rely on visual inspection and x-rays, neither of which can reveal the true nature of soft tissue dysfunction.

Myofascial Release is a very powerful technique allowing us to treat soft tissue dysfunction which does not respond to other methods at our disposal. As with any method of treatment, Myofascial Release should not be used exclusively for the treatment of our patients. It is another method of approach, an adjunctive treatment which gives us still another weapon in our arsenal, allowing us to remove the pain from our patients' bodies.

Many therapists have been using soft tissue mobilization methods for years without placing that name on what they are doing. The philosophical difference between soft tissue mobilization and Myofascial Release lies in permitting and encouraging patients to be equal participants in the process of removing restrictions from their bodies. As you become skilled in this technique, the feedback from patients becomes very consistent and very positive. Comments like "How did you know that's where I hurt?" or "That's exactly where it hurt when I twisted my ankle" or "I had forgotten about that. How did you know it was there?" occur repeatedly. Once you begin receiving this type of feedback from patients, there will be no question that Myofascial Release as a technique is accurate, useful and effective.

How to Use This Manual

The purpose of this manual is to teach the technique of Myofascial Release as a mechanical skill first. The anatomy of the myofascial complex is described before each technique. Since the sensation of relaxation is magnified through the long levers of the arm and leg, the Arm Pull and the Leg Pull are the first skills presented. Once you have learned to recognize the sensation of relaxation through touch, the rest of the single therapist techniques are presented. Multi-therapist techniques are presented next because they require the same level of expertise in terms of the initial learning process. The advanced techniques of Treatment in Three Dimensions, Trigger Point Releases and Releasing the Dural Tube require the most skill in responding to patient feedback. These cannot be learned until you are able to work entirely from feedback and therefore, are presented last.

Only after you have learned the skills do you need to learn the somewhat unique assessment which I use. I believe the assessment makes more sense when viewed from the standpoint of what postural changes can be achieved by Myofascial Release. The transition of this mechanical technique into a therapeutic art is that intangible change to which all therapists must aspire. It is the difference between therapists and the difference between their effectiveness in applying these principles of treatment. This change comes with practice of the skill and with the application of the "people skills" we all use.

Significance of Touch

Touch is powerful. Some people believe that touch can heal. Historically, touch is the basis of much of what we do as physical therapists. Some, however, have become afraid of touching their patients for fear of being accused of not being scientific or professional. Insurance companies want quantification of progress and refuse payment for treatments that cannot be measured on a machine. The effect of touch cannot be measured with a goniometer or strain gauge. The effect of touch is measured as a subjective sensory experience.

Touch teaches us to recognize thickness and form.[12] It is the earliest sense to develop in the embryo.[13] The infant's first communication with the world is through touch. A baby learns the world is a safe place when it is held and cuddled.

The first feel of our bodies comes from the touch of our parents. The amount of affection we receive in the pre-verbal period of life has a significant influence on how we feel about ourselves and on our self-esteem in later life.[14] In Rene Spitz's classic study, institutionalized children who received good physical care but were deprived of touch failed to thrive.

The adult who has experienced touch as a pleasant, comforting sensation in the past will come into physical therapy wanting and expecting to be touched. The association of touch with pleasure facilitates the healing process. The adult who has had positive touch experiences in the past has no problem recognizing present touch as therapeutic and helpful. Treatment with any of the manual therapies is accepted and welcomed. This adult brings positive expectations into treatment and is able to work with the therapist toward the therapeutic goal.[15] The adult who has experienced touch as abusive in the past will come into physical therapy expecting and dreading touch, but not necessarily with any conscious awareness of this. This person is constantly on guard and is unable to fully relax. He is much more comfortable with the modalities than the therapist.[15]

At some point in everyone's life touch becomes sexualized. For the fortunate, this occurs around puberty. This individual can easily distinguish between sexual and non-sexual touch, albeit some choose not to! This person can also convey touch as either sexual or non-sexual.[15]

For those who have been sexually abused, sexualization of touch occurs with the abuse. This individual consciously or subconsciously associates touch with abuse and with sex. Similarly, the individual who has been physically abused consciously or subconsciously associates touch with physical abuse. If these associations are conscious, psychotherapy can help the individual change his perception of touch to a more accurate perception of present touch. However, if this association is subconscious, the individual has no way to access these memories and to learn to more accurately interpret the meaning of present touch. This individual will react to present touch as though it is the same as the past negative touch. Thus, the patient's responses will be "off" without the patient or the therapist having a clue where these responses are coming from.[15]

Dissociation allows the individual to emotionally and mentally leave his body when verbal or physical touch becomes too threatening to tolerate. Dissociation occurs along a continuum with daydreaming at one end and multiple personality disorder at the other. Dissociation is a valid and valuable defense mechanism which allows an individual to survive intolerable conditions. However, once learned and used, dissociation may be used indiscriminately in all situations of (perceived) intimate contact whether or not the situation is, in reality, a threat.[15]

The past experiences of both the therapist and the patient in terms of touch and perception of present touch help determine the therapeutic milieu. Either or both could dissociate with touch. If the dissociator is the therapist, the patient will feel a coldness and emptiness in the therapist's touch. If the dissociator is the patient, the therapist will feel unresponsiveness, coldness and emptiness in the patient's body. Unless the therapist is aware of this dynamic, the entire experience can be misinterpreted and result in a mislabeling of the patient's problem.[15]

The therapist's role is to define the therapeutic relationship. Through touch within well-defined boundaries, the therapist conveys competency, compassion, and trustworthiness. When dealing with an individual who has difficulty trusting, keep in mind that trust is *always conditional*. Trust is fragile and must be earned by the therapist at each visit with every patient regardless of the length of the therapeutic relationship.[15]

A Communication Exercise

When you place your hands on your patient, your mind should be clear of distracting thoughts and chatter. If you are planning your grocery list or reviewing a conversation you had previously, you cannot be open to the patient you are supposed to be working with. This inattention will be translated to your hands. To prove this to yourself, try this exercise with someone you trust. Make up some notecards with the following instructions, one to a card.

1. You have just had a fight with another person (not me) and are very angry.

2. It is a beautiful day and you are very happy.

3. You are bored.

4. You have a zillion things to do and want to get this finished quickly.

5. You are very tired.

6. You are jumpy.

Shuffle the cards face down. Have the other person take a card, read it, and respond to it while holding one or both hands on some part of your anatomy acceptable to you. Then write down what your response is to that feel. Compare your responses to what your partner was trying to convey after you have gone through all the cards. You may want to have a third person act as timer and hold each sensation for one to two minutes.

General Instructions for Myofascial Release

There is nothing written in concrete about Myofascial Release techniques. It is a forgiving technique, one which you can easily adapt to take advantage of your strengths. You use the positions which are the most comfortable and efficient for you. For the initial purpose of teaching, I use my favorite positions. There are no absolute right or wrong ways to perform this technique—just different ways. Be forgiving of yourself as you learn and have an open mind. Myofascial Release is different from any other stretching technique you have ever learned. Join me on this journey and I hope you enjoy it as much as I do.

To learn the techniques that follow, you must be relaxed and able to focus on the feedback coming through your hands. The ease with which you learn Myofascial Release techniques depends upon how far you can allow yourself to relax into sensing and experiencing your patient's body through your touch. Relaxation is the key—if you are tense or wound up, you will not be able to feel through your own tension. If you are tense, you will be unable to feel the inherent tissue motion which is vital to guiding this technique. Your patient will feel your tension and be unable to relax. Some of your patients will be so tense that they are unable to recognize the sensation of relaxation until you teach it to them. So, before trying to learn Myofascial Release you must teach yourself to relax if you have not already done so. The first step is developing your own body awareness. There are many ways to do this—from relaxation imagery to Feldenkrais to Myofascial Release itself. Cultivating a permissive attitude toward yourself is essential to the development of body awareness. If you are continually questioning or criticizing yourself, you will block feeling your own body responses. You need to put aside your judging mind and focus inward, becoming aware of your body as you stand, move, sit, breathe and stay still.

The key to learning Myofascial Release is to listen to the messages and sensations within your own body. If you can learn to monitor your feelings, you will gain far more than if you mechanically imitate the techniques presented here. Try to use a "beginners" mind, coming to each technique openly, spontaneously, without preconceptions, expectations and goals. Be childlike. Take each technique as an exploration or adventure to be experienced. Stay in the fullness of the moment, trusting your own experience to bring what you need to learn.

Develop a capacity for sustained awareness or attention in order to be able to perceive and respond to the sensory messages from your body. Train your awareness, heighten your ability to be fully present, and learn to quiet your rational mind. The observing mind has a broader view which comes forward when the rational mind quiets down.

Quieting your rational mind means watching your thoughts without identifying them. If you pursue them or criticize them, you disturb your concentration more. The more you can lessen the hold of your rational mind, the more you will be aware of and in touch with the numerous subtle sensory messages sent and received within your own body.

I have used a variety of techniques to teach the sensation of relaxation to my students and my patients. There are a lot of relaxation audiotapes which are available commercially. Sometimes I will make personalized tapes using language which is more meaningful to that individual and focusing on specific body parts which are more tense than others. In my experience, relaxation tapes which instruct you to tense a body part and then relax are more useful than those which just instruct you to relax. People who have trouble relaxing need to be taught the contrast of tension and relaxation. Feldenkrais lessons teach the sensation of relaxation using indirect methods.

When I began using these techniques, I worked in a darkened room illuminated by small night lights, thinking this would help my patients relax. I no longer do this on a routine basis. I found that some of my patients became scared. Ultimately, I learned that these patients were dealing with memories of abusive events from the past. It is out of the scope of this text to discuss handling these abuse memories. I would urge the reader interested in learning more about dealing with abuse memories to read *Craniosacral Therapy and Somato-Emotional Release: The Self Healing Body*.[16]

Others equated the atmosphere created by the night lights with so-called new age treatment. Some liked this sensation while others were distinctly uncomfortable. This was not the atmosphere I wished to convey to every patient. Once I am familiar with my patient, I may choose to work in a darkened room if it allows him to be more comfortable and relaxed. The only patients with whom I consistently work in a darkened room are those with severe and/or migraine headaches. These individuals are usually light sensitive and will request the lowered lighting. As a general rule, I work with normal lighting in my treatment rooms in part to keep the atmosphere and boundaries of my relationship with my patient very well defined.

Regardless of the light level, I ask my patients to close their eyes and to focus all their attention on the sensations within their bodies. Then, I ask that they focus very narrowly on the sensation of my hands on their body. Finally, I ask that as their attention begins to wander (because it will just as mine will sometimes wander) that they re-focus on the sensations in their body beneath my hand or hands. There are two reasons for giving these instructions. The most obvious is the spoken instructions telling my patients what they need to do as their part of the treatment. The other is to give permission (in a way) to my patient to be less than perfect, while acknowledging and affirming how difficult it is to stay focused all the time. Many people with whom I work function on the "should" level, as in "I should stay focused," "I should be good," "I should exercise every day," and "I should be perfect." With my instructions I attempt to show that there are no "shoulds" in my treatment.

Most of the time I work with my eyes closed. This has not been a conscious decision to do so, but is a pattern which has evolved for me. Initially, I worked with my eyes closed to force myself to attend only to the sensations under my hands. Otherwise, I was more likely to find myself trying to analyze what was happening between my patient and me. Therefore, I found it necessary to rely only on what I could feel and not what I could see. Interestingly, psychologists tell us that when there is a conflict between what you hear and what you see, you will believe what you see. I would further expand that concept and say that when there is a conflict between what you see and what you feel, you will believe what you feel. The resolution of these conflicts can be very difficult to achieve (see Assumptions, pages 3-5). It is out of the scope of this text to go into a detailed discussion of this conflict. However, I would hope that the serious student of Myofascial Release would pursue further study of psychology for this information.

There is a significant body of literature on the difference between right brain and left brain functioning. Different ways of thinking and functioning have been ascribed to the right or left brain based upon research on the localization of functions in the hemispheres. Left brain functioning is described as rational, logical, linear and verbal. Right brain functioning is described as irrational, illogical, nonlinear and nonverbal, i.e., relying upon sensations. In reality we are all "ambi-brained." In some situations we work in left brain mode and in others we work in right brain mode.

As a therapist, knowing how you function most effectively should help you develop a treatment style in which you are the most comfortable.[17] As a therapist, do you consider yourself a helicopter pilot who sees the whole forest or a pathfinder who sees the trees?[18] Are you most comfortable telling your patient what to do and designing complete exercise programs? Or do you prefer to wait for and respond to your intuitive response to your patient's problem? Someone who is most comfortable and most effective functioning in a left brain mode may not be as comfortable using Myofascial Release. The right brained individual may find that Myofascial Release meshes with his preferred mode of functioning.

In summary, Myofascial Release is a right brain mediated stretching technique which uses the sensation of touch to convey acceptance of the patient as the patient currently is and to facilitate change which the patient wants. The technique is permissive in the sense that there is no right or wrong way to react to the gentle stretching. The patient's responses guide the stretching, showing the therapist what to stretch, in what order to stretch and how to stretch.

The Process of Change

Initially, do not expect the response to the stretch to last. Explain this transient nature of change to your patient to prevent him from assuming blame for a supposed "failure" to improve. Postural change is mediated in the central nervous system which must be re-educated to accept and maintain this more energy efficient posture. Myofascial Release disrupts the individual's homeostasis. I always warn my patients that initially they will feel worse as muscles must learn to function in different ways. Balance is altered as posture becomes more symmetrical. Initially, the central nervous system recognizes the old posture as more comfortable and familiar while the new posture is more painful and strange. Gradually, as posture changes, the central nervous system recognizes the new posture as more energy efficient, but still painful and unfamiliar. As the new posture becomes less painful, it is maintained more consistently. Finally, the central nervous system recognizes the new posture to be more energy efficient and comfortable while the old posture is less efficient and painful.

A partial explanation of the mechanism of Myofascial Release can be found in the following physical laws. A fuller explanation awaits the researchers' ability to quantify what we, as clinicians, already see. For the time being we can only speculate on the mechanism of Myofascial Release. Clinically, significant postural changes can be documented as the result of Myofascial Release, but to date, no peer-reviewed research studies have been published. Unfortunately, this holistic treatment technique does not lend itself to clear-cut research with definitive results. In contrast to other stretching techniques, the therapist using Myofascial Release does not set out to stretch one myofascial group using one specific technique. This makes comparison studies extremely difficult to construct.

According to the Law of Facilitation, when an impulse has passed through a set of neurons to the exclusion of others, it will tend to take the same course on future occasions. Each time this path is traversed, resistance to stimulation is smaller. The Law of Facilitation explains why you never forget how to ride a bicycle.

This law also explains why it is so difficult to change habitual posture even when a different posture is necessitated by physical changes to the body. For example, after insertion of Harrington rods, patients will complain of feeling off-balance and of trying to return to their original distorted posture. Until the patient adjusts to this enforced posture, she will have difficulty walking a straight line and will complain of feeling like she is going to fall.

The Arndt-Schulz Law tells us that gentle touch increases physiologic activity while heavy touch is inhibitory. Myofascial Release uses both types of touch depending upon the needs of the patient. Light touch and light stretching encourage relaxation. Light touch also allows the therapist to ease into areas of tightness without triggering reflex muscle guarding. As gentle stretch promotes progressive relaxation of tight structures, deeper restrictions can be accessed and treated. Gentle stretch does not inhibit the excessive micro-contraction present at active myofascial trigger points. Heavier pressure is needed to inhibit the muscle spasm which perpetuates the trigger point.

Once the nerve centers are stimulated, the stimulus is carried throughout the body in accordance with the Law of Diffusion. There is no way to affect one area of the body without affecting the entire person. For example, once past childhood, Americans do not participate in nonsexual hand-holding. Good boundaries between patient and therapist will allow recall of this nonsexual contact, facilitating those childhood feelings of security, protection, caring and trust. Therefore, when beginning to stretch the palm of the hand or using a hand hold for stretching of the upper quarter, a variety of emotional responses may be triggered in the patient. All are necessary preconditions to allow the patient to feel comfortable with his responses to myofascial stretching.

In contrast, the Law of Avalance states that multiple sensations may be aroused in the brain by a simple stimulus in the periphery. Many feelings and responses may be aroused by any peripheral stimulus. We need to be aware of the effect we have upon our patients just by the simple act of touching them in a caring, sensitive, accepting, open manner. From the first moment I touch my patient I am conveying a message which may or may not be accurately interpreted by my patient. I cannot emphasize too strongly the need for the therapist to have well-defined boundaries and the ability to verbally define those boundaries in a nonthreatening manner to the patient.

An Overview of Treatment

Once the evaluation or assessment is completed, then you can decide which area is to be initially targeted for treatment and how the patient is to be positioned for the beginning of the treatment. No matter which area of the body I initially plan to treat, the first thing I do is sit quietly with my hand or hands cradling the back of my patient's neck or resting on his shoulders. As I am quiet, I am able to feel my patient's natural body rhythm and can also feel in which body areas that rhythm is disrupted. If there are multiple areas of disruption, I will begin with the one which feels the most superficial.

I visualize myofascial restrictions using Fritz Perls' onion metaphor. The most superficial restrictions must be released before the next layer can be accessed. The process is repeated for each layer until the deepest restrictions can be reached for treatment. What happens if you make the wrong choice of where to begin the stretch? The worst case scenario is that the myofascial unit will tighten up again and you get another chance to find the most superficial restriction. Do not confuse this with the seesaw response of the entire body as the central nervous system is re-educated to accept a more symmetrical posture. When you have decided where to begin stretching, lay your hands on that area and gently palpate the area using your entire hand. As you detect your patient's inherent body rhythm, the specific area of restriction within that myofascial unit will be felt as both tension and altered rhythm. You may wish to palpate more deeply with your fingertips until you locate the taut bands of the myofascial trigger points.[19] However, this degree of specificity is not necessary prior to beginning treatment. In fact, I rarely palpate for the taut bands until after I have completed at least one or two treatments aimed at the more superficial restrictions and trigger points. I find it necessary to locate the taut bands only when I get to the level of fine tuning and treatment of the deeper restrictions.

Next, gently stretch the targeted tissue between your hands along the direction of the line of the muscle fibers until a resistance to further stretch is felt. Hold this position until the soft tissues relax, releasing the excess tension which was maintaining the malalignment.

If your patient has been able to remain focused on the sensations immediately beneath your hands, he will recognize this release as a relaxation and lengthening of the entire area. Maintain your contact at all times. After the initial release of tension, further releases may occur without any change of your contact. This may be felt as waves of movement flowing throughout the area or as stepwise releases with definite beginnings and ends. When no further release of tension is felt, again stretch the tissues between your hands to take up the slack and hold this new elongated position. The process is repeated until the tissues are in a fully elongated position or until an end feel is reached.

The above describes the essence of Myofascial Release. Whether or not you are treating your patient in two dimensions or three dimensions, the underlying stretch is always the same. Whether or not you are focusing on one muscle or myofascial unit or the upper quarter of the body, the underlying stretch is always the same. Whether or not your patient is lying quietly on the treatment plinth or exhibiting spontaneous movement, the underlying stretch is always the same.

As the restrictions are peeled away layer by layer, your patient may relive the event which resulted in her injury. If her response to that injury was not fully experienced at the time, she may have repressed the memory and have no conscious knowledge of the injury. She may experience a flashback causing her to re-experience the injury as though it were happening in the present. If this re-experiencing results in your patient now having conscious memory of the event, she has experienced a physically facilitated abreaction.[15] This has been called a somato-emotional release by Upledger.[20]

Freud described abreactions as bringing to conscious memory that which was repressed with all of the sensations, behavior, affect and knowledge of that event. While psychotherapists facilitate abreactions verbally, physical therapists can do this nonverbally through touch. It is out of the scope of this manual to present an adequate discussion of physically facilitating abreactions.[16] Physical therapists should not purposely facilitate abreactions unless the therapist has an extensive background in psychology and counseling. Merely revivifying the memory is abusive. A thorough processing of the memory and integration of the memory is necessary for a positive therapeutic outcome.[15]

Myofascial Restriction and the Anatomy of Fascia

The following conceptual models are offered to assist in the visualization of myofascial restrictions for the therapist who is just beginning to use Myofascial Release. As you become more comfortable and proficient using Myofascial Release, you will probably find this visualization unnecessary.

Imagine all of the fascia in the body to be a continuous air-filled balloon with "out-pouching" which houses the various organs and muscles. If part of the balloon cannot expand enough to allow the part which it is covering to be housed easily, the rest of the balloon must accommodate by shifting toward that part. This, in turn, causes another part to be crowded by the balloon's walls, necessitating another shift. When no further accommodation can be made by the balloon, the parts must be compressed by the immobile wall of the balloon, causing significant postural asymmetries. Obviously, the better solution to this compression is to stretch the balloon's walls to accommodate the structures which need to be inside.

Looking at the same balloon, it is obvious that a distortion on any part will be felt throughout the continuous skin of the balloon. The smallest tug or pull will move the entire balloon toward that force just as the smallest puff of wind will push it away. Thus, there is no way to affect only one part of the balloon.

Another way to view the fascia in the body is to consider it as a large square sheet of plastic wrap. This square fully covers the entire body. If the plastic wrap is pinched or is stuck on itself, the sheet can no longer be a square and will no longer cover the entire body unless the body twists and folds to fit under the altered shape of the sheet. Until the sheet is smoothed out again, it cannot fulfill its function of covering the body while permitting symmetrical posture.

Picture a skeleton with tight red plastic overlays depicting the muscles and fascia. As the overlays are stretched, white stress lines appear and the skeleton's shape must change to keep the overlays attached to it. In order to visualize what is happening in the body when tightness or restriction is present, imagine the latissimus dorsi on the right side of the skeleton and the quadratus laborum on the left. Fully flex the right humerus, retract the right shoulder and protract the right side of the pelvis. The left side of the pelvis must retract and the lumbar spine must rotate. Picture the stress lines in the quadratus laborum as the left side of the body is rotated to the right.

Pick any other two muscles and place them on the skeleton. Put one of the muscles on its maximum stretch, then visualize the resultant stress on the other muscle. This game can be played over and over with the same result each time, showing that any myofascial restriction at, near or far from a target muscle causes distortions not only in the target muscle but in other muscles as well. Thus, all myofascial restrictions must be treated and released to restore proper alignment and energy-efficient movement to the entire system.

Fascia has been regarded as extraneous tissue without consideration that it might have a distinct function all its own. As Garfin, et al.[21] state: "The functional relationships between fascia and the forces and pressures generated by the underlying muscular contractions are poorly understood." Few research projects have studied the biomechanical effects of fascia on muscle or explored the effect that removal of the fascia has on the underlying muscle and osseofascial compartment.[21] In the medical model, when severe fascial restriction occurs, the fascia is removed without consideration of the additional biomechanical consequences the loss of fascia might produce. In fact, fascia assists in maintaining muscular force by controlling muscle pressure and volume. The effect of fasciotomy is a 15% loss of muscle strength.[21] Myofascial Release, an alternative to removal, is frequently capable of decreasing myofascial constriction and the accompanying pain, diagnosed as compartment syndrome, without compromising muscle strength.

Few anatomy texts show fascia other than as a structure to be removed to expose the more important organ systems. Cailliet,[11] in contrast, lists fascia as a type of connective tissue along with tendons, ligaments, cartilage, muscle and bone. In a schematic drawing of fascia, the fascia is actually divided into three layers. The **superficial fascia** or hypodermis lies beneath the dermis and consists of loose connective tissue and adipose tissue. The dermis is connected to the subcutaneous layer by fibers extending into the superficial fascia. In turn, the superficial fascia is attached to the underlying tissues and organs.[22] The superficial fascia provides storage for water and fat, serves as insulation, prevents and protects from mechanical deformation, and provides a pathway for nerves and blood vessels.

The second layer is called a **potential space**. This space may enlarge with extravasation or edema, suggesting that the fascia can be disrupted and stretched by any injury, no matter how minor. The **deep fascia** is a dense sheet or band of fibrous connective tissue which separates the muscles into functioning groups and which lines the body covering all organs of the body. The function of the deep fascia is to allow free movement of the muscles, fill the spaces between the muscles and other organs, provide passageways for the nerves and blood vessels, and in some instances to provide attachments for the muscles. Fascia itself is essentially avascular. Surgical incisions are often made where the fascia overlaps or is fused. The strength of these areas allow for firm anchoring of sutures and secure wound healing.[22]

The **epimysium, perimysium** and **endomysium** are extensions of the deep fascia. This continuous fibrous connective tissue divides and surrounds fasciculi and ultimately each muscle fiber. These three divisions of fascia may extend beyond the muscle cells to form tendons or aponeuroses attaching muscle to muscle or muscle to periosteum.[22]

Individual muscle groups are enveloped by fascia separating one muscle group from the next. Fluid between the fibers of the fascia acts as a lubricant, allowing free movement of one muscle past another. Bursae are formed in some areas between muscles, between muscles and either tendon or bone, or beneath the skin over bony prominences.[11, 23, 24]

The connective tissue fibers that form the fascia are arranged approximately in one plane to form membranes. The fibers run in various directions so that they appear interwoven with no one direction predominating. This is in contrast to tendons, in which fibers run roughly parallel to each other.[23] Because the fibers in fascia run in all directions, fascia is distensible in all directions to accommodate changes in muscle bulk and to permit stretching. Fascia shrinks when it is inflamed. It is slow to heal because of a poor blood supply; it is a focus of pain because of its rich nerve supply.[11]

Testing for Vascular Integrity

Before beginning any treatment, assessment of your patient's vascular status should be a part of your regular routine. Begin with your patient sitting.

Compression of the brachial artery can be detected by taking the radial pulse in both arms, and compression of the subclavian artery can be detected by performing Adson's test[25] (Figure 1). Unequal pulses or ablation of the radial pulse with head rotation can be caused by soft tissue compression, bony compression and/or vascular disease. Depending upon your findings, you may choose to perform further tests of vascular sufficiency. In addition, you may want to measure blood pressure in both arms.

With your patient supine, gently palpate the carotid pulses *one side* at a time with the head in the midline position. Simultaneous palpation can provoke a carotid reflex or syncopal attack (Figure 2). The pulses should be roughly equal in strength.[25] If you detect a significant difference in the strength of these pulses, you may want to refer your patient

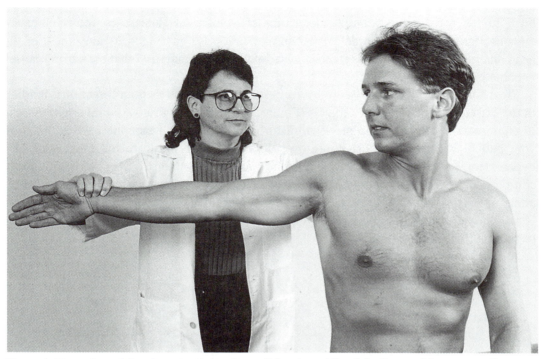

Figure 1. To perform Adson's test palpate the radial pulse while abducting and hyperextending your patient's arm as he rotates his head to the same side. The test is positive if ablation of the pulse occurs.

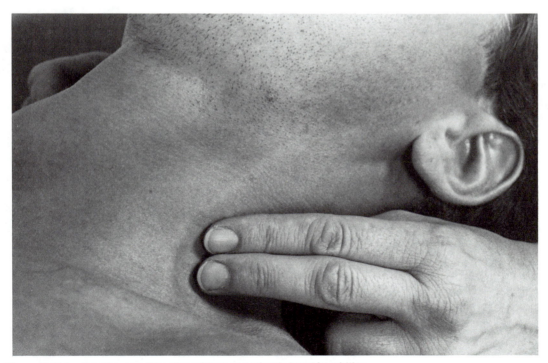

Figure 2. Palpating the carotid pulse with your patient's head in midline.

back to his regular physician to determine if Myofascial Release is contraindicated. Unequal carotid pulses are a definite contraindication for any vigorous movement of the head and neck. As soft tissue restrictions are released, you may find that the carotid pulses become more equal in strength.

Test for vertebral artery disease by fully rotating the neck in both directions, holding in the extreme range for a few seconds (Figure 3). The patient with vertebral artery disease or compression will complain of visual disturbances and light headedness. Next, position your patient with his head extending over the edge of the plinth to place his neck into hyperextension (Figure 4). Dilation of his pupils is another sign of vertebral artery compression.[26] Since soft tissue compression of the vertebral arteries can mimic vertebral artery disease, the above are not absolute contraindications for Myofascial Release. However, you may choose to refer your patient back to his regular physician before beginning treatment.

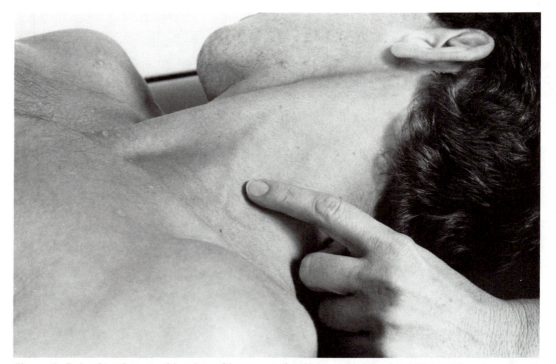

Figure 3. Palpating the carotid pulse with your patient's head in lateral rotation while observing for symptoms of vertebral artery compression.

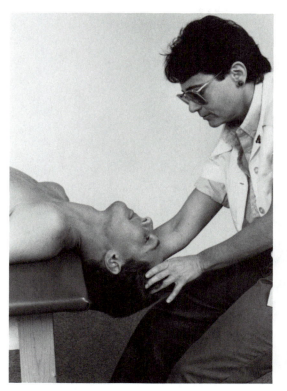

Figure 4. Observing pupillary response to neck hyperextension to detect vertebral artery compression.

Impaired circulation to the lower extremities can be detected by checking the femoral pulses (Figure 5), popliteal pulses (Figure 6) and either the dorsalis pedis (Figure 7) or the posterior tibial pulses (Figure 8). Absence of the femoral pulse is a contraindication for treatment of the lower extremity and requires further evaluation by the patient's physician. In contrast, absence of the other pulses can be due to soft tissue compression mimicking vascular disease. You may choose to refer your patient back to his regular physician if you cannot palpate these pulses after several treatment sessions. It is imperative to continue to monitor your patient's pulses throughout the course of treatment when you have identified soft tissue compression.

Setting the Stage

Once I have completed my initial assessment, I no longer ask my patients to disrobe for treatment. When I was first learning Myofascial Release, I needed the extra feedback of having my hand directly on my patient's skin. Now I can feel the inherent body motion even through clothing. If I have a patient who prefers to wear a shirt, I do ask that she wear one with an open or loose neck. I explain that I do not want to stretch her clothing or create a feeling of being strangled. If I anticipate deep releases in the lower extremities, I ask my patient to wear shorts. Some of my patients prefer to wear loose jogging clothes or sweat suits while others are comfortable removing their shirts.

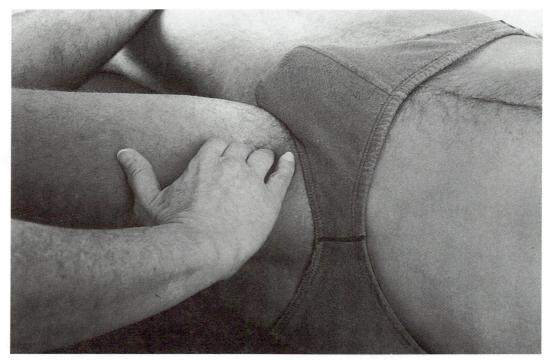

Figure 5. Palpating the femoral pulse.

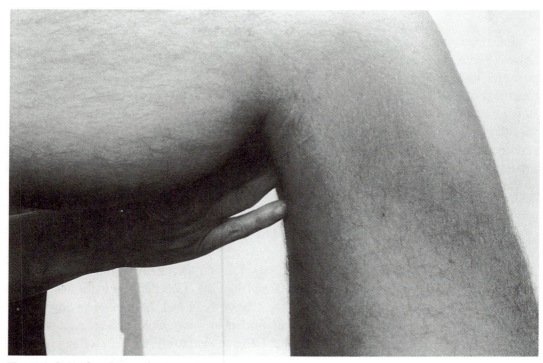

Figure 6. Palpating the popliteal pulse.

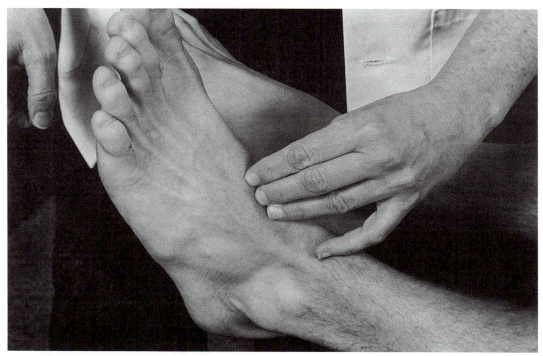

Figure 7. Palpating the dorsalis pedis pulse.

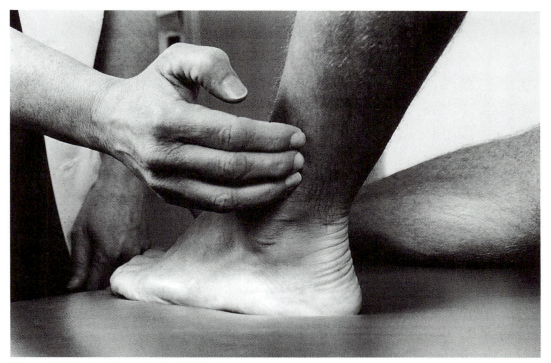

Figure 8. Palpating the posterior tibial pulse.

Most of the time I work alone. When I work with a man, initially my assistant is in the room throughout the treatment time. When I work with a woman, I rely on my intuitive response during the initial interview to determine if I want my assistant in the room. I do not permit family members or others in the treatment room because this may inhibit my patient's response to treatment.

I do ask my patients to remove all jewelry, take off their belt and loosen any tight clothing prior to beginning treatment. I also remove my watch to avoid accidentally scraping my patient with it. If you wear rings or a bracelet, you should remove them as well. I have given up wearing belts to avoid accidentally injuring my patient as I move about. I found that removing my belt in front of my patient was frightening to some. If you wear a belt, you may want to remove it prior to entering the treatment room.

Treatment should begin with the patient and therapist in proper position. Both for learning purposes and for initial treatments, I ask my patient to lie supine on the plinth. Your forearms and elbows should rest on the plinth next to his head (Figure 9). Your treatment stool must be at a height that places your arms at an angle which allows relaxation of your shoulders. Improper height of your treatment stool will cause your shoulder muscles to be too tense to allow efficient movement.

You need to be in a comfortable position and able to use good body mechanics rather than muscle power. Relying on strength will overpower the inherent tissue motion and will exhaust you. Maintaining a light touch while staying loose and relaxed will allow you to feel refreshed after using Myofascial Release all day.

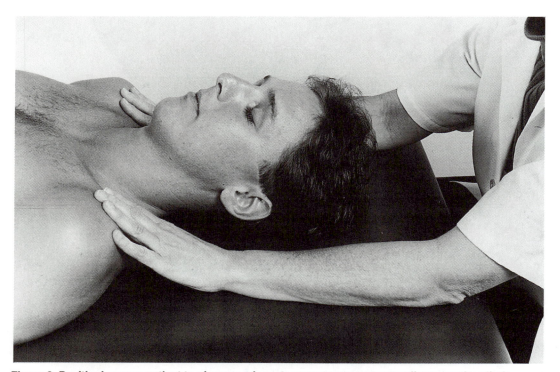

Figure 9. Positioning your patient to give you adequate room to support your elbows on the plinth.

If you are tall, you may need to bend your knees during some stretches to avoid stressing your low back, or you may choose to sit on a mobile stool or lean against a wall. Having a treatment plinth which is the right height for your comfort is very helpful. If you are short, you may need to stand on a riser or stool. Once again, having a plinth scaled to your height is the best long term solution. But no matter what the height of the plinth, you will have different requirements depending upon which stretch you are doing.

I have at least one broad low riser on which I can stand next to each one of my plinths. In addition, I have a mobile stool set for my height. Sometimes I will sit on the plinth next to my patient, and sometimes I will kneel or stand on the plinth next to my patient. Each of my treatment rooms is set up slightly differently so I can choose the one which is best for the treatment I anticipate doing. Do whatever you need to do to position yourself for comfort and efficient movement.

Drink...Drink...Drink...Drink...Drink

While removing restrictions to efficient movement, Myofascial Release also causes waste products to be released from the tight structures. These waste products must be flushed from the patient's body or your patient will complain of increased pain and overall body aches. Some will complain of having flu-like symptoms.

You cannot rely on your patient's natural thirst to cause him to drink adequate fluids. I tell my patients to drink a minimum of one additional gallon of fluid on the day of treatment and one to two days afterward. This fluid should be low in sugar, low in caffeine, and non-alcoholic. Fruit juices, decaffeinated coffee and tea, artificially sweetened soft drinks and water are best. I encourage my patients to drink water primarily.

As the therapist you may find yourself having some of the same symptoms as your patients if you do not drink extra fluids. When you first start using Myofascial Release, you may find yourself thirsty all the time. Why does this happen? My hypothesis is that as you treat your patients you relax your own excessive tightness, releasing metabolic waste products. Obey your body's message and increase your fluid intake. You should increase your fluid intake by one additional gallon per day whether or not you are thirsty. As you become more experienced, you might not require as much fluid.

Be Kind to Your Hands

Many Myofascial Release techniques result in compression of the finger joints and in overall hand fatigue. Decompression is achieved by loosely gripping each finger between your thumb and first finger and stroking the length of each finger in turn (Figure 10). Decompression should be performed periodically during each treatment session and at the end of each treatment session. This stroking decompression can also be used with your patients for both the fingers and toes. Stroking decompression of your toes is something nice you can do for yourself too.

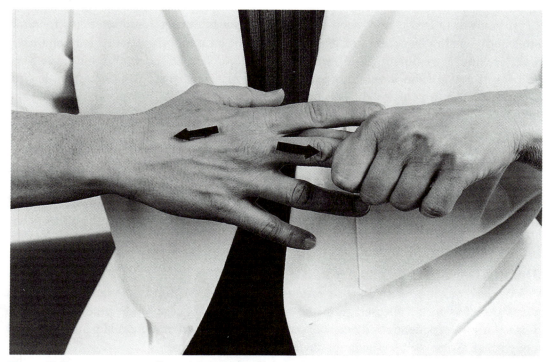

Figure 10. Decompress your finger joints periodically during and after every treatment session.

II

Basic Myofascial Techniques

Fascia of the Arm and Shoulder Regions

The superficial fascia of the arm and shoulder contains a variable amount of fat. Superficial nerves and blood vessels run through both the superficial and deep fascia. The tough membranous layer of brachial fascia encloses the muscles of the arm, forming a sheath completely around the arm. This sheath is loose-fitting anteriorly to allow bulging with muscle contraction. Posteriorly, the fascia is fused to the flatter triceps brachii muscle. Medially and laterally, the fascia is attached to the humerus, forming the medial and lateral intermuscular septa.[23, 24]

In addition to containing a variable amount of fat, the superficial fascia in the pectoral region encloses the glandular breast tissue. The superficial fascia is not well developed in this region and is most often fused with the deep fascia. The fascia divides and splits to surround each structure in the pectoral region and then reunites to form a single layer again. It is attached to the bony prominences and also gives attachment to some of the fibers of the underlying muscles. Suffice it to say, each muscle has its own fascial coat. [23, 24]

Stretching the Upper Quarter–Arm Pull

Stand next to your patient's side so that you can comfortably grasp your patient's hand and maintain your own relaxation. Move toward your patient's feet, placing traction on the arm by pulling downward toward his feet in line with the fibers of the deltoid muscles (Figure 11). Use just enough traction to counterbalance your patient's arm so you are supporting his arm completely.

Initially, your patient's hand will either be pronated or in a neutral position. Grasp your patient's hand, with one hand holding the hypothenar eminence and the other hand holding the thenar eminence. Do not hold with your fingertips but use your thenar eminences, spreading your patient's palm and reversing the usual concave posture of the palm (Figure 12). With this hold you can stretch the interosseus muscles and the palmar fascia while stretching the entire upper quarter. Slowly rotate the forearm into full supination. If you feel any resistance to this movement, back off slightly and wait for relaxation to occur before moving into more supination. Repeat this sequence until no further supination is available.

Many people will give you very positive feedback to this specific hand grip. It feels very good to have the palm stretched, releasing tension that is rarely recognized or felt until contrasted with relaxation.

Now gently increase the amount of traction until you feel a slight amount of resistance. Maintain the traction, focusing all of your attention on the feedback you are receiving through your hands, and wait for the soft tissues to relax. As they relax you will feel a gentle give of the entire arm. Apply a little more traction to take up the slack and wait again for a release to occur. Continue doing this until an "end feel" has been reached, indicating that the arm is stretched as far as it can be in that position at that time. An end feel is the sensation of no further stretching being available.

Check that your shoulders and arms are relaxed. If you have become tense during this process, consciously relax and see if you still have an end feel. If you no longer sense an

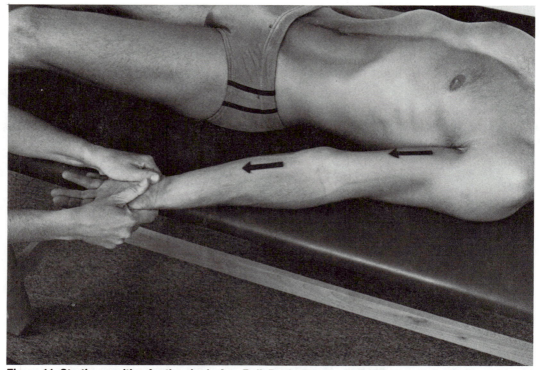

Figure 11. Starting position for the single Arm Pull. Begin the Arm Pull with your patient's arm at his side in external rotation so that his thumb points to the direction of movement. Apply traction in line with the fibers of the deltoid.

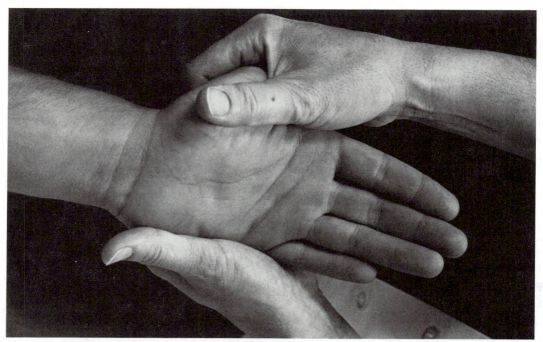

Figure 12. Stretching of the interossei by gripping your patient's hand on the thenar and the hypothenar eminences using your fingers as a fulcrum on the back of his hand. As the palm is slowly stretched laterally and downward, the normal concave posture will initially flatten and end in a slightly convex position.

end feel, apply a little more traction to your patient's arm and repeat the sequence again until the end feel is again reached.

It is very important that you understand the need for relaxation and attention to feedback for you to successfully learn the techniques of Myofascial Release. Therefore, once you have reached an end point, ask your patient to cross his legs. What happened to what you were feeling? Did you lose the feedback you were getting? Do you feel more tension or a sensation of twisting? How did this feel to your patient? Sometimes a release will occur with this movement of the legs, although not necessarily from actually crossing the legs but rather from the shift of focus and the deep breath your patient takes as the movement is performed.

Now have your patient tense his crossed legs and feel again how much more tension is present in his arm. Next have your patient tighten up his crossed legs and then relax. Feel the increase followed by a decrease in tension flowing through your hands. How did this feel to your patient?

Have your patient relax and uncross his legs. Now tense up your arms and shoulders. What happened to what you were feeling? Did you lose the feedback you were getting? Tension in you will override what you can feel from your patients. Now consciously relax again. What happens? Does the feedback return? How does this feel to your patient? Tension throws "noise" into the system and prevents the kinesthetic link from occurring. Repeat this exercise as many times as you need to until you can quickly catch yourself or your patient becoming tense.

Let us perform one more exercise before returning our full attention to the Arm Pull. Return your attention to the feedback you are receiving from your patient. Now ask the patient to focus his attention elsewhere, perhaps on planning what to have for his next meal. What happens? Does your feedback disappear? Does it feel like your patient left the room? Now ask your patient to return his attention to your contact. What happens? Does your feedback return? While your patient stays focused on your contact, let your attention wander. What does that feel like to you? To your patient?

At this point, all of the muscles with fibers running parallel to the trunk should be in their fully elongated position. Now, very slowly begin to abduct your patient's arm, maintaining external (lateral) rotation (Figure 13). If you feel any resistance or roughness of motion, back off slightly and wait for the feeling of relaxation before abducting further. As you do that, part of the range of motion is going to feel like you've just "grooved in." This is a feel of smoothness and rightness of position. Everything feels to be in balance. It is at this point in the range that your patient is able to move most efficiently and with the least energy expenditure. It is this feeling we are trying to reproduce throughout the entire range of motion. As you leave this part of the range, resistance or drag with be felt again. As before back off slightly, pause, wait for a release and then continue slowly leading the arm into more abduction if the arm is not already starting to lead you into that position. The arm may begin to move spontaneously at any point in the range of motion. If that occurs, follow the motion, placing just enough drag on the arm to keep the movements slow. This will allow you to feel hesitations or restrictions. When one is felt, stop the motion and wait for a release before allowing the motion to continue.

If your patient is trying (subconsciously) to avoid tightness or pain, his arm may begin to move very quickly through the range of motion. You must stop this movement and take

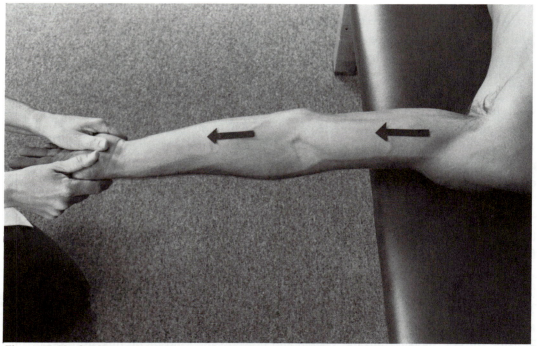

Figure 13. Moving into abduction during the single Arm Pull. If the arm does not spontaneously move into abduction, gently and slowly abduct the arm while maintaining traction and continuing the Arm Pull. As tightness or hesitations are felt, stop the motion, maintain the traction and wait for the tissues to relax before continuing the abduction. Do not allow the motion to continue through any tightness.

his arm back to that part of the range just before the painful or restricted arc. Go very slowly into this range of motion and wait very patiently for the release to occur. For the purpose of learning this technique, if you cannot release this area in a fairly short period of time, skip over it by allowing some shoulder flexion to occur. However, in a real treatment situation, you will not want to progress any further in the range until this painful arc is fully relieved.

If you have a patient with a pathological condition around the shoulder joint, in the anterior chest wall or in the parascapular region, you will reach a point at which it just does not feel right to continue. Back off a few degrees, hold that position and wait. If no further releases occur, you may want to switch to mobilization techniques or terminate the active part of the treatment session.

Continue to bring the arm around into full abduction, slight flexion and rotation until the elbow is proximal to the ear (Figure 14). Maintain this position of stretch until an end feel is reached. Once again check to see if you have become tense during this movement. If you have, consciously relax and determine if you still have an end feel. If you do not, increase your traction slightly and wait for the relaxation to occur. Continue until no further relaxation can be obtained.

While maintaining the same amount of traction on your patient's arm, bring the arm into 90 degrees of flexion and abduction stretching into scapular protraction. You will want to change your hand grip and/or your body position for this maneuver. Maintain an upward traction as you wait for the muscles of retraction to relax and release the scapula

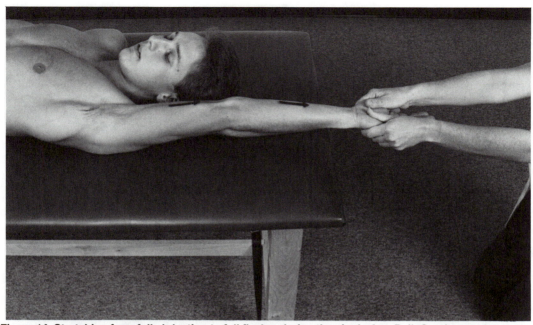

Figure 14. Stretching from full abduction to full flexion during the single Arm Pull. Continue to follow the spontaneous movement until the arm is next to the ear. If your patient does not have full range of motion at the shoulder joint, you may need to allow some flexion at the shoulder joint.

to move into full protraction. If you feel the retractors pulling back strongly, rather than trying to overcome them with more traction, push the arm back into retraction. When you feel the retractors release, again apply traction moving into protraction. You may want to apply traction to your patient's arm with your upper hand while leading the scapula into protraction with your lower hand (Figure 15).

Once full protraction has been achieved, begin to lead your patient's arm into horizontal adduction. Once again go slowly, waiting for the releases to occur until an end feel is reached. This can be the end point of the Myofascial Arm Pull. If you choose to stop, gently lower your patient's arm back to his side and the forearm across his abdomen. If full relaxation of the upper quarter has occurred, the arm will have a heavy relaxed feel similar to the feel of an infant or young child who has fallen asleep on your shoulder.

Another way to stretch the protractors of the scapula is to continue bringing the arm across the body from a fully extended position, rolling your patient onto his opposite side. As your patient rolls, apply traction to your patient's hand or arm with one hand. Place your other hand at the medial border of the scapula and lead the scapula into protraction (Figure 16). If you feel the scapula pull back strongly, change your traction force to compression into the shoulder joint and stabilize the scapula with your other hand (Figure 17). When you feel the retractors of the scapula relax, resume traction and protraction. The scapula will release and ride forward on the rib cage until it is fully protracted. As described above, the arm will feel very heavy and relaxed. Allow your patient to roll back to supine and rest the fully relaxed arm on his body.

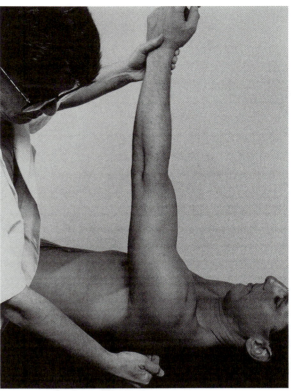

Figure 15. Leading the scapula into protraction with your patient's arm flexed and adducted to 90 degrees.

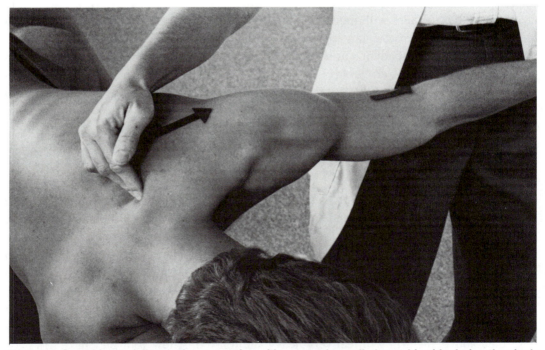

Figure 16. Stretching to full scapular protraction with your patient rolled onto his side during the single Arm Pull. Once full abduction is achieved in the frontal plane, continue to follow or lead the arm into horizontal adduction across the patient's body with your lower hand, while distracting and protracting the scapula with your other hand. The arm continues to be externally rotated throughout this motion.

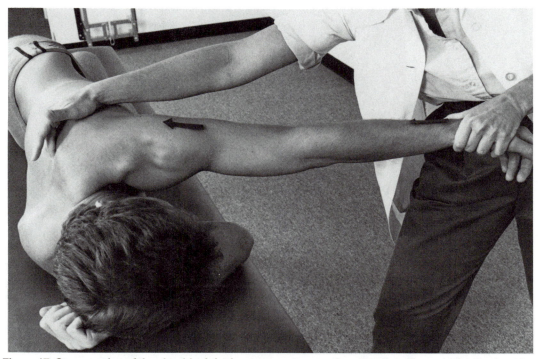

Figure 17. Compression of the shoulder joint in response to scapular retraction. If your patient's shoulder begins to retract spontaneously, compress the shoulder joint and retract the scapula by pushing the arm back into the joint and releasing your distraction at the medial edge of the scapula. When relaxation of the scapular retractors occurs, resume traction on the arm and protraction of the scapula.

Two motions of the shoulder joint have not been addressed at all by the Myofascial Arm Pull with your patient supine–internal rotation and hyperextension. External rotation has been only partially addressed. I prefer to address rotation by abducting the upper arm to 90 degrees and flexing the elbow to 90 degrees. Maintain traction with one hand just above the elbow joint while your other hand guides the arm into rotation (Figure 18). Once again slowly move through the range of motion until resistance or drag is felt. Back off slightly, wait for the release to occur and continue to move through the range of motion. Tightness of the pectorals may need to be addressed before full range of rotation can be achieved.

Hyperextension of the shoulder joint can occur as a natural part of the motion if, at 90 degrees of abduction, the arm is led into hyperextension. Your patient must be positioned close enough to the edge of the plinth to allow this motion (Figure 19). Hyperextension is more easily addressed by performing the Myofascial Arm Pull with your patient in the prone position.

Specific handgrips are not a part of the Myofascial Arm Pull. The heart of this technique is responding to the feedback from your patient, as felt through your hands. If you have a patient who for some reason is not comfortable with the hand hold described above, you can shift your grip to above the wrist (Figure 20), to the mid-forearm (Figures 21 and 22) or to above the elbow (Figure 23).

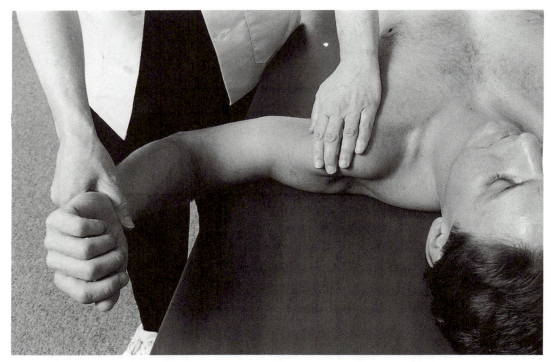

Figure 18. Stretching into shoulder external rotation while stabilizing your patient's shoulder joint.

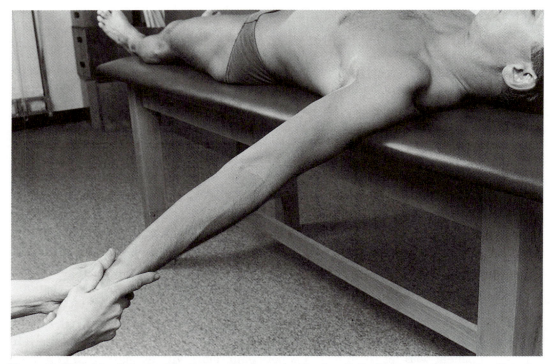

Figure 19. Stretching into shoulder hyperextension using the Arm Pull with your patient supine. Note the model's increased lordosis and hip and knee flexion indicating inadequate relaxation prior to posing for this stretch. If this occurred during an actual treatment session, you would need to return to straight plane stretching until your patient's back and leg were more relaxed.

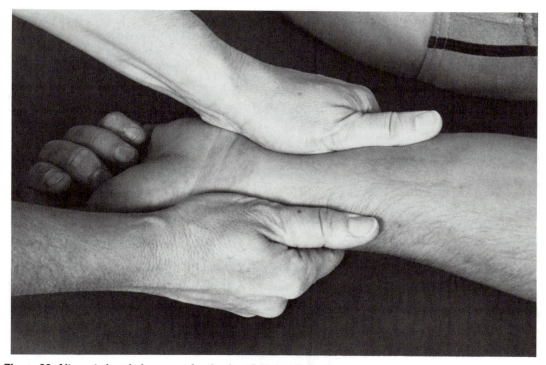

Figure 20. Alternate hand placement for the Arm Pull, holding above the wrist. If your patient experiences wrist or hand pain due to your handgrip during the Arm Pull, he will be unable to relax and allow full stretching of the upper quarter. The pronator quadratus can be stretched at the same time with this handgrip.

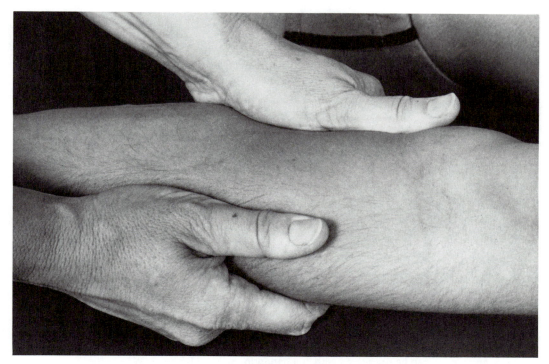

Figure 21. Alternate hand placement for the Arm Pull, holding in the upper portion of the forearm. The pronator teres can be stretched at the same time with this handgrip.

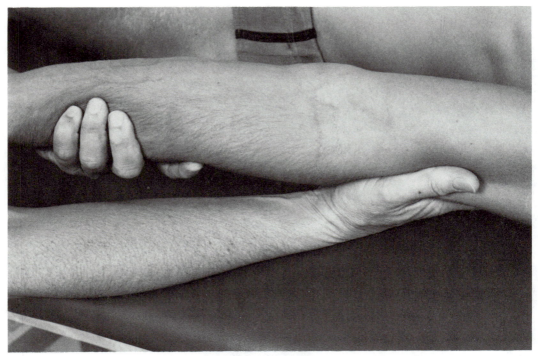

Figure 22. Alternate hand placement for the Arm Pull, holding above and below the elbow.

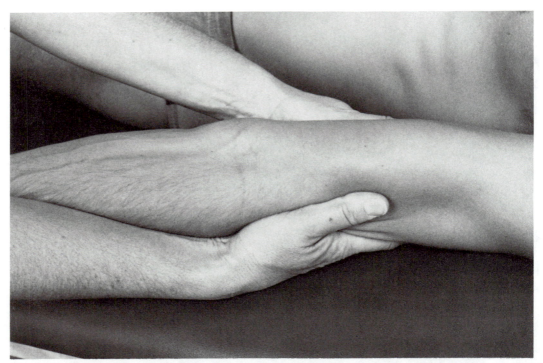

Figure 23. Alternate hand placement for the Arm Pull, holding above the elbow. Crossed fiber stretching of triceps and biceps can be performed with this handgrip.

You can use any hand hold that is comfortable to you and to your patient and that achieves the objective that you and your patient set for that treatment session. Always keep in mind that the objective is often set and achieved with nonverbal communication. Using a hand hold that either you or your patient finds to be uncomfortable is counterproductive and negates the entire treatment session. Both of you must be relaxed.

During the Myofascial Arm Pull you may sense that a muscle does not "know" when it should relax. The muscle may be constantly in a tense state and not "recognize" this state as undesirable. A very simple way to focus attention on this muscle is to place one hand on the tense muscle and apply light traction (Figures 24 and 25). Your immediate feedback if you have made the correct assumption is relaxation of the targeted muscle.

If a myofascial trigger point is preventing full relaxation, there is a very different feel to the muscle. In this case you will feel the muscle relaxation stop at the trigger point. No matter what angle of approach you use, you keep coming back to that same spot. It is possible to treat the trigger point at the same time as the Myofascial Arm Pull.

Trigger Point Releases are addressed on pages 123-127. It is important to learn the basic techniques of Myofascial Release first, before adding Trigger Point Releases. Trigger points may be released during the simpler process of stretching and may not require specific attention later. Thus, maximum stretch should be achieved at all points in the range of motion before any Trigger Point Releases are attempted.

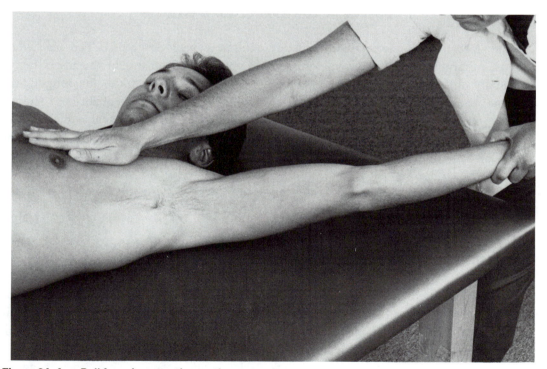

Figure 24. Arm Pull focusing attention on the pectorals.

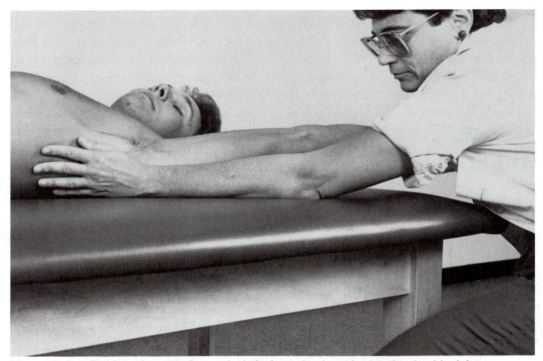

Figure 25. Arm Pull focusing attention on the latissimus dorsi proximal to the shoulder joint.

Fascia of the Lower Extremities

The fascia of the lower extremities is extremely well developed. The fascia lata encloses the posterior hip musculature and the muscles of the thigh. The fascia lata is especially strong on the lateral border of the thigh where it includes the longitudinal iliotibial band. Strong intermuscular septa extend on each side of the quadriceps femoris muscle, attaching to the femur. Medially, septa border the adductor canal, which houses the femoral artery as it extends into the popliteal space. Cylindrical fascia enclose the lower leg musculature with septa on each side of the peroneal muscles attaching to the fibula. A transverse septum separates the deep and superficial calf muscles. The lower leg fascia holds the tendons that pass from the leg to the foot, where well-developed fascia exist on the dorsum and in the sole of the foot.[23, 24]

Stretching the Lower Quarter–Leg Pull

With your patient in the supine position, cup his heel in one hand while dorsiflexing his foot with your other hand and maintaining his hip in full extension (Figure 26). Hold his foot in this neutral position, place traction on his leg to counterbalance its weight, and wait for the release to occur. Once the initial release has occurred, increase your traction to take up the newly available slack. Wait for the release and increase your traction again. Continue to repeat this process until an end feel is reached. At the end point, no further relaxation will occur and his leg be fully extended.

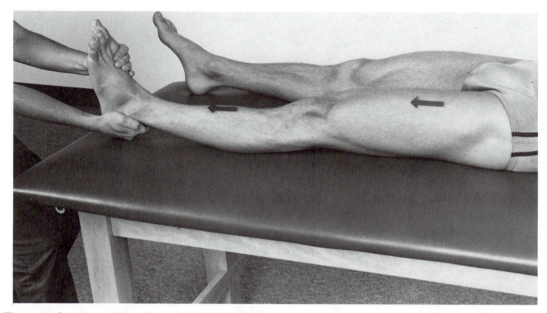

Figure 26. Starting position for a single Leg Pull with the foot held in a neutral position. The patient should not be actively dorsiflexing his foot to neutral, but should be held in neutral by the therapist.

Externally rotate his leg as far as your patient can permit while maintaining his hip and knee in full extension (Figure 27). If full external rotation is not achieved, maintain your traction and rotate his leg until tightness is felt. Back off a few degrees, hold until a release occurs, take up the slack, and repeat this process until an end feel is reached.

Once full available external rotation is achieved, if spontaneous abduction has not already begun, gently move his leg into abduction (Figure 28). Move slowly so that you may feel any hesitation or tightness in the range of motion. When you feel a hesitation or tightness, stop, back up a few degrees, and hold until a release occurs. Repeat until you reach an end feel. Maintain hip distraction throughout the range of motion.

When full abduction is achieved in the sagittal plane, flex his hip while maintaining traction to allow distraction of the pelvis (Figure 29). Treat the pelvis the same as the scapula. Place your lower hand under his buttock and lead it forward while tractioning his leg with your upper hand.

Depending upon your size and strength relative to your patient, you may need to stand on a riser or even on the plinth to apply enough traction to stretch the gluteals in this fashion. If the hip starts to retract, reverse your force to compress into the joint. Wait for the release and distract again. Once full distraction is achieved, allow his leg to cross midline causing him to roll onto his side (Figure 30). Continue distracting his hip to further stretch the buttock muscles. At this point, his leg may move into full extension again or into further hip flexion. If his leg begins to move spontaneously, follow the motion while maintaining just enough drag to keep the motion slow. When a restriction or hesitation is felt, stop the motion, back up a few degrees, if necessary, and hold until a release occurs. Repeat until an end feel is reached.

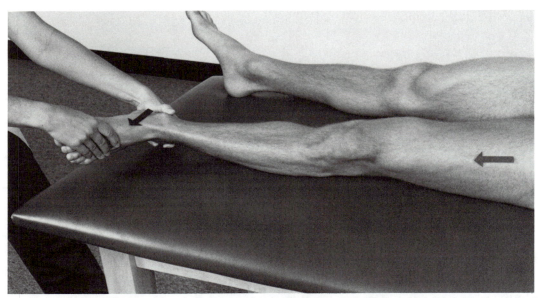

Figure 27. Stretching into external rotation during a single Leg Pull. While maintaining traction, slowly move your patient's leg into external rotation using his foot as the lever.

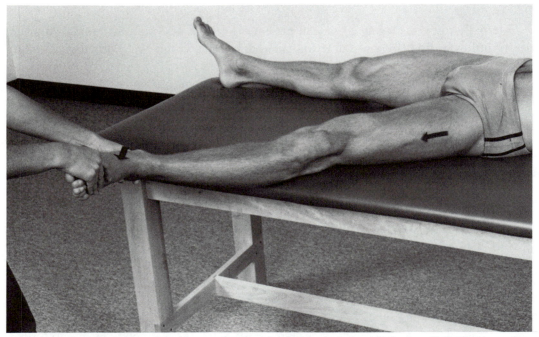

Figure 28. Stretching into abduction and external rotation during a single Leg Pull. Once maximum external rotation and traction are achieved, bring your patient's leg slowly and gently into abduction if spontaneous abduction does not begin. Follow or guide his leg to full abduction, repeating the same movement with the leg as was described with the arm.

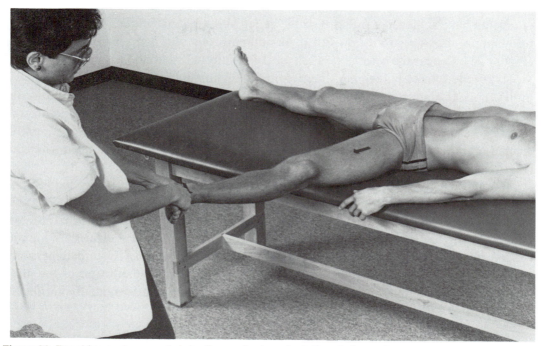

Figure 29. Reaching end range of abduction and external rotation during a single Leg Pull. The amount of abduction available will vary greatly from patient to patient. Only through the proprioceptive feedback from your patient will you know when the maximum is reached.

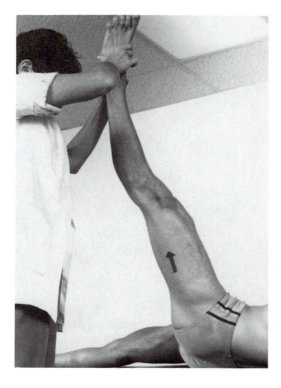

Figure 30. Horizontal adduction and external rotation of the leg and protraction of the pelvis during the single Leg Pull. When full abduction is reached, guide the leg into horizontal adduction, while maintaining traction on the leg. This will bring the pelvis into protraction as the hip is both flexed and adducted to 90 degrees.

If you have achieved a full stretch of the leg and hip musculature with your patient on his side, move his foot into full inversion and rotate his leg into internal rotation (Figure 31). Repeat the release process until full internal rotation is achieved or an end feel is reached. Lead his leg back across midline while maintaining traction and pelvic protraction. If his hip pulls back into retraction, exaggerate the movement by pushing his leg into his hip joint (Figure 32). As relaxation occurs resume traction and protract the pelvis as he rolls onto his back. Continue to retrace the circle with his leg internally rotated until his leg is once again adducted to neutral with full hip and knee extension (Figure 33).

If your patient has a pathological condition at the hip joint, full range of motion may not be achieved. Should spontaneous movement occur, there is no need to continue through the full Leg Pull because the patient will be showing you which restrictions need treatment. Because you are responding to the feedback from your patient through your hands, you will not exceed the safe range of motion for your patient. If your patient cannot tolerate the pressure of your hand at the ankle (Figure 34) or dorsiflexion of the ankle (Figure 35), any alternate handgrip or position may be used that is mutually acceptable (Figure 36).

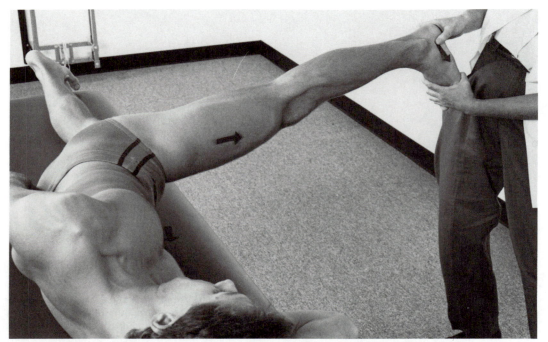

Figure 31. Beginning of the reverse single Leg Pull with the leg adducted and internally rotated. When full horizontal adduction is complete, slowly place the leg into internal rotation, waiting for any tightness to be released before proceeding. Retrace the arc of motion, releasing any tightness as it is located until the leg is back in the starting position.

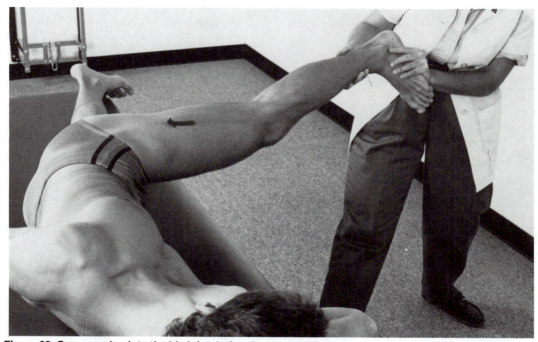

Figure 32. Compression into the hip joint during the reverse single Leg Pull. If the pelvis begins to retract, compress the hip joint in the same manner as you would the shoulder joint, wait for the release and resume traction again.

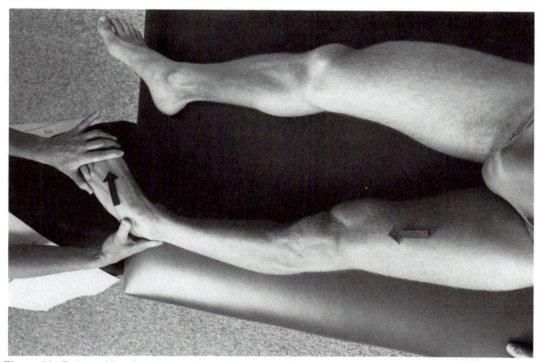

Figure 33. End position for the reverse single Leg Pull. Note that the model has very limited internal rotation. He is trying to substitute forefoot adduction for internal rotation.

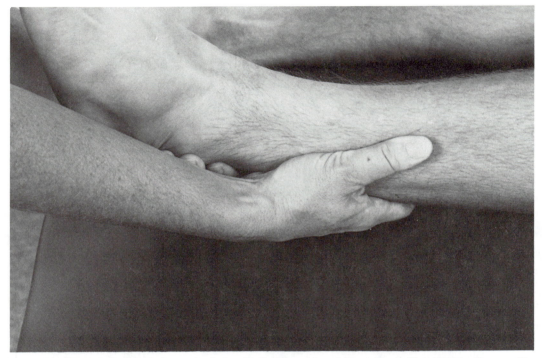

Figure 34. Alternate hand grip for a single Leg Pull with one hand above the ankle and the other cradling the calcaneous.

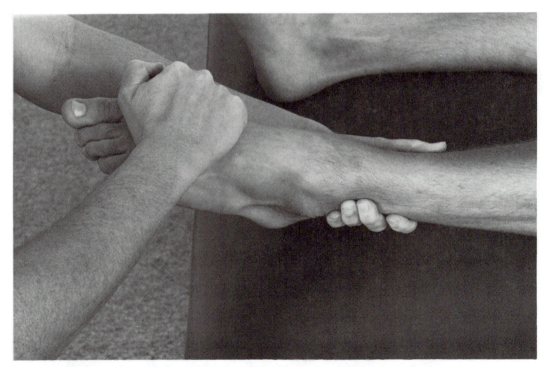

Figure 35. Alternate hand grip for a single Leg Pull with the foot held in plantarflexion.

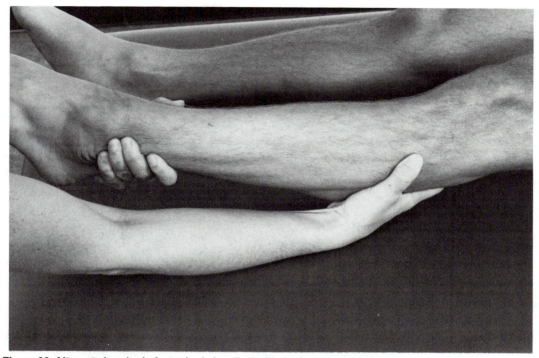

Figure 36. Alternate hand grip for a single Leg Pull with the hands widely spaced on the lower leg avoiding traction on the ankle joint.

Focused Stretching of Specific Muscles

Any muscle or myofascial unit that allows the placement of two hands or even two fingers can be stretched to relieve myofascial restrictions. One hand or finger acts as the anchor from which the stretch originates. The other is used to provide the stretching force. Alternately, body weight can be used as the stabilizing force, freeing the therapist's hands to provide the counterforce at two different places at the same time.

Hand and body placement should be comfortable for both you and your patient. For large muscle groups such as the erector spinae (Figure 37), the middle trapezeii (Figure 38), or the quadriceps femoris (Figure 39), you may gain better leverage by crossing your hands. For small muscles like the masseter, only one or two fingers are needed (Figure 40).

Place one hand or finger proximal to the distal attachment of the muscles to be stretched, using just enough pressure to stretch the superficial skin and fascia and to stretch the underlying muscle(s) in the direction of the muscle fibers. The downward pressure used to anchor the myofascial unit being stretched should be firm. If too light a touch is used, the unit will not be adequately anchored. The patient will interpret this as ineptness on the part of the therapist. There is no way to quantify the proper amount of anchoring pressure for each myofascial unit for individual patients. The therapist must learn from feedback how to grade this pressure and assume it will change over the course of treatment. As treatment progresses to deeper layers, the anchoring pressure will change as will the stretching pressure.

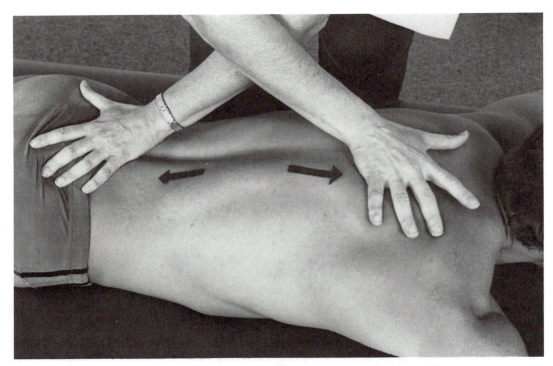

Figure 37. Cross-hand longitudinal stretching of the lumbar and thoracic erector spinae.

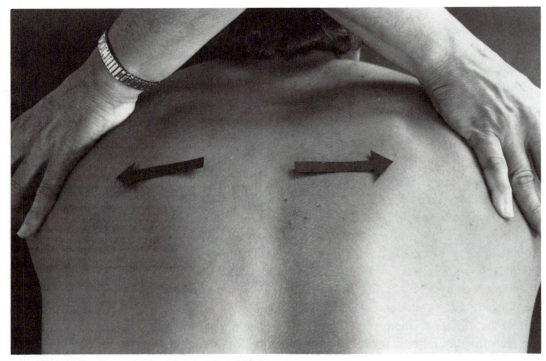

Figure 38. Cross-hand longitudinal stretching of the middle trapezii.

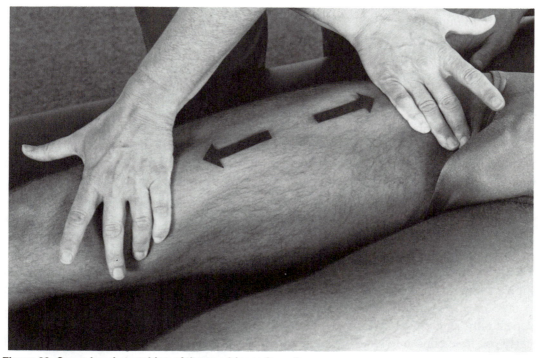

Figure 39. Cross-hand stretching of the quadriceps femoris.

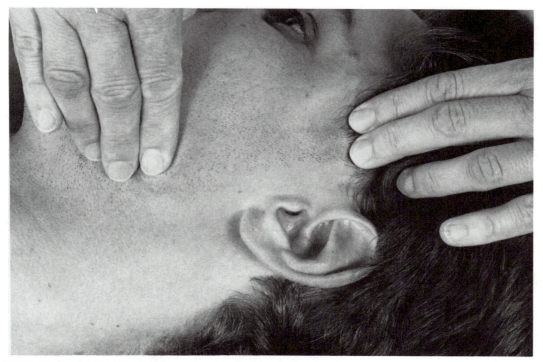

Figure 40. Stretching the masseter using two fingers of each hand.

Hold this position until all of the soft tissue is felt to relax, then stretch again, taking up the additional slack created by the release. Repeat this process until an end feel is reached. Slowly and gently release your stretch pressure and re-evaluate for restrictions and rebound tightening.

Erector Spinae

The erector spinae can be stretched in segments roughly reflecting its separate sections, or it can be treated as one long muscle. Crossing your arms will allow you to push against the muscle with your stronger muscles (see Figure 37). This will be less fatiguing than using uncrossed arms and stretching with your shoulder abductor muscles.

Firmly anchor one end of the erector spinae using the ulnar border of your hand, pushing downward and outward parallel to the muscle fibers. I like to stand on a low riser to gain better leverage. Place your stretching hand on the other end of the section of the erector spinae you have chosen to stretch, pushing downward and outward at the same time. The amount of downward pressure should be adequate to prevent your hand from slipping and dictated by feedback from your patient's body. Use enough outward stretch to take up the available slack. Hold until the soft tissues relax and then stretch again. Repeat until an end feel is reached.

If you have chosen to stretch the erector spinae by sections, leave your anchoring hand in place and move your stretching hand up to the next section. Repeat the stretching sequence again until an end feel is reached. Continue moving section by section until the entire length of the erector spinae has been stretched. While no further relaxation can be achieved using this technique, further relaxation may be achieved using a two or three person technique which will be described later. Fine tuning of the stretch will be described in Section III, *Advanced Techniques*.

Upper Trapezii

With your patient lying supine, sit behind his head with your forearms resting beside his head. Place your hands on his upper shoulders keeping your elbows straight and using your body weight as the stretching force (Figure 41). Your patient's body weight acts as the stabilizing force. Push your hands downward and outward at the same time so the scapulae are placed in a neutral position in regard to protraction and retraction. As you push downward and outward, take up the available slack. Wait for the soft tissues to relax and stretch again. Repeat until an end feel is reached. Initially, you will be stretching the shoulder portion of the upper trapezii, but as the available slack is taken up, your patient will report feeling a stretch in the neck portion also.

Shoulder Portion of the Upper Trapezius

If you wish to remain seated or standing at your patient's head, shift to the side you want to stretch. Stabilize at the base of his neck using either the ulnar border of your hand (Figure 42) or the web space. Place the ulnar border of your other hand proximal to the shoulder joint and push outward toward the shoulder joint. Wait for the soft tissues to relax and stretch again. Repeat until an end feel is reached. You can also stand or remain seated by your patient's side. Place the web space of your stabilizing hand against the base of his neck and the ulnar border of your other hand proximal to his shoulder joint (Figure 43).

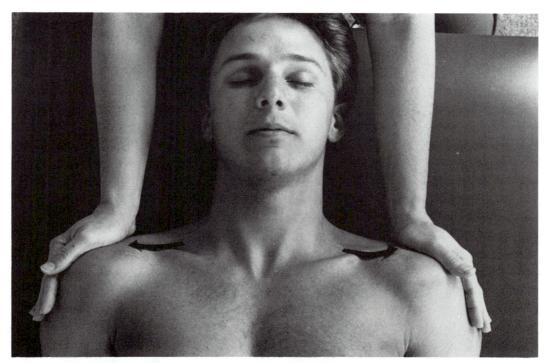

Figure 41. Bilateral stretching of the shoulder portion of the upper trapezii. Note that the direction of stretch is downward and outward at the same time.

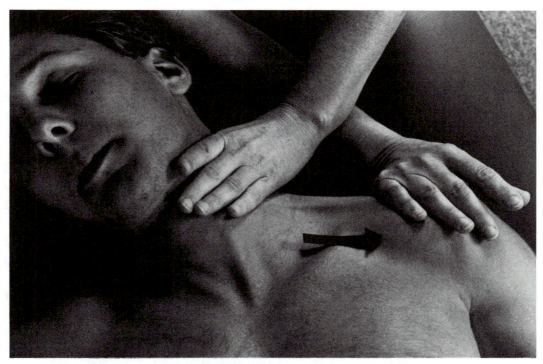

Figure 42. Unilateral stretching of the shoulder portion of the upper trapezius with the therapist at the patient's head.

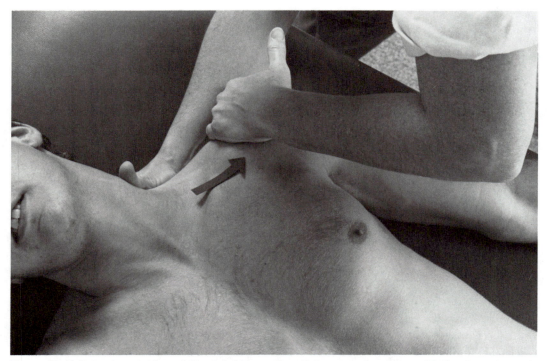

Figure 43. Unilateral stretching of the shoulder portion of the upper trapezius with the therapist at the patient's side.

Pull his shoulder toward you to take up the available slack. Wait for the soft tissues to relax and stretch again. Repeat until an end feel is reached.

Neck Portion of the Upper Trapezius

The neck portion of the upper trapezius will be stretched during stretching of the posterior cervical musculature. Sometimes you will need to focus on the neck specifically to stretch the scalenes along with the neck portion of the upper trapezii. This can be performed as a unilateral or bilateral stretch depending upon which technique is chosen.

Sitting at your patient's side, cup the mastoid process in the web space of your hand while using the web space of your other hand to stabilize at the base of his neck. Apply enough distracting force to take up the available slack. Wait for the release and repeat until an end feel is reached. If spontaneous movement begins, apply enough drag on the movement to allow you to feel any skips or hesitations. When this happens, stop the motion until a release occurs and then allow the motion to resume. Continue until an end feel is reached.

Alternately, you can sit at your patient's head and place the outer border of your thumbs against the mastoid processes. Apply traction by extending your fingers against the base of his neck (Figure 44). Once you have taken up the available slack, wait for the soft tissues to relax and stretch again. Repeat this process until an end feel is reached. If spontaneous movement begins, apply enough drag on the movement to allow you to feel any skips or hesitations. When this happens, stop the motion until a release occurs and then allow the motion to resume. Continue until an end feel is reached.

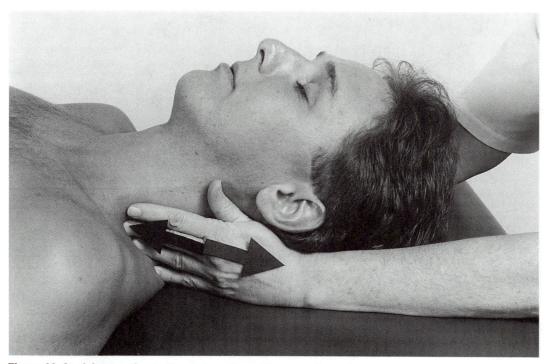

Figure 44. Applying traction to the neck portion of the upper trapezius.

Middle Trapezii

With your patient lying prone, stand in front of his head and place the ulnar border of each of your hands at the distal attachments of the middle trapezii. Once again, you will be more energy efficient by crossing your hands to use a pushing force rather than using uncrossed hands and using your shoulder abductors. Use just enough downward force to keep your hands from sliding off of his back. Use enough stretching force to take up the available slack and wait for the soft tissues to relax. Increase your force to stretch again and repeat until an end feel is reached.

Lower Trapezius

The lower trapezii are more often over-stretched by persistent tightness of the upper trapezii and the elevators of the scapulae. However, at times you may need to stretch the lower trapezius to free up scapular motion or to allow you access to the deeper layers of the back. You can use the ulnar border of both your hands or the ulnar border of one hand and the base of the palm or any other combination which you find comfortable. Place each hand firmly at either end of the lower trapezius (Figure 45). Use enough downward and outward force to keep your hands from slipping and to take up the available slack. Wait for the soft tissues to relax and stretch again. Repeat until an end feel is reached.

Pectorals

The pectoral muscles can be stretched from a variety of positions. You can reach these muscles easily whether you are at your patient's side or head. Since the muscle is relatively small, you can be equally efficient stretching with your hands crossed or uncrossed.

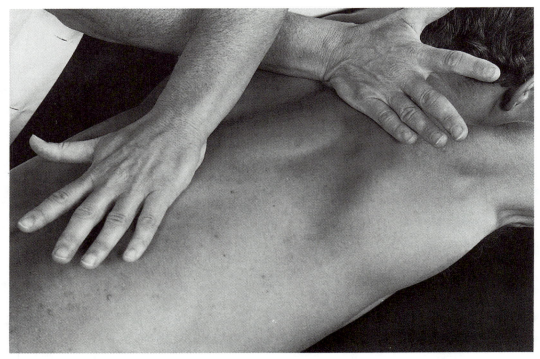

Figure 45. Stretching the lower trapezius.

The pectoralis major has two distinct portions which must be approached as different muscles for a maximum stretch to be achieved. The upper set of fibers runs parallel to the clavicle and responds to stretching in a straight lateral fashion. The lower fibers of the pectoralis major fan from the ribs and sternum up to a point where they join the tendon as it inserts into the humerus. The pectoralis minor must be stretched after the more superficial fibers are relaxed.

When your patient exhibits full protraction of the scapulae, strengthening the muscles of scapulae retraction is needed in addition to continued stretching of the pectorals. Unfortunately, most exercise machines at health clubs encourage strengthening of the pectorals but not the upper back. Therefore, I ask my patients to stop using those machines and to strengthen the upper back muscles, emphasizing the scapular retractors until a better balance is achieved.

Horizontal Fibers of the Pectoralis Major

To begin stretching the upper portion of the pectoralis major, place both hands on the muscle, gently stretching medially and laterally across the horizontal fibers (Figure 46). Hold until it releases and stretch again. Continue until an end feel is reached. If the horizontal fibers will not stretch any further and an end feel has not been reached, you may need to release the diagonal fibers before the horizontal fibers will relax completely.

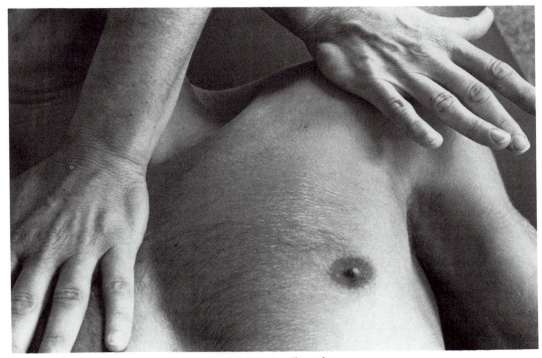

Figure 46. Stretching the horizontal fibers of the pectoralis major.

Diagonal Fibers of the Pectoralis Major

Once the horizontal fibers have been stretched, direct your attention to the fanning fibers below them and change the angle of your stretch (Figure 47). You may want to move your hands down only one to two inches, taking the remainder of the muscle in small sections depending on how much of the muscle you can cover with your stretching hand. As each section releases its excess tension, you can widen the area between your hands. Keep your stabilizing hand proximal to the shoulder joint while stretching downward on a diagonal to take up the available slack. Wait for the release to occur and stretch again, continuing on the same diagonal until the full length of this section of the muscle is stretched. Continue until an end feel is reached. Then move back upward and stretch the next section of fibers which you could not initially cover with your hand. Repeat until the entire diagonal portion of the pectoralis major has been stretched.

Once the entire muscle is stretched in sequential fashion, spread your hands to cover as much of the muscle at one time as possible for a final stretch. This will tell you if any restrictions remain in the muscle and allow you to focus your attention on any remaining myofascial restriction.

Pectoralis Minor

As the pectoralis major relaxes, tension in the pectoralis minor can be felt. You will recognize the pectoralis minor by the direction of the tension. Allow the tension to guide your hand placement. Initially, you may need to keep a mental image of the pectoralis minor to help direct your stretching.

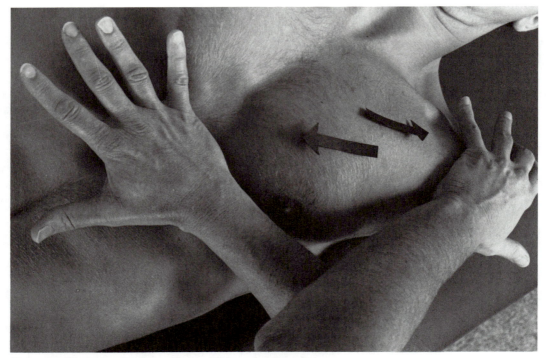

Figure 47. Stretching the lower fibers of the pectoralis major.

Move your stabilizing hand to the attachment of the pectoralis minor and let the heel of your stretching hand apply the traction. Wait for the release and stretch again. Repeat until an end feel is reached.

When no further tension is felt beneath your hand, both the pectoralis major and minor are in their fully elongated position.

Arm Pull

Focusing on the Horizontal Fibers of the Pectoralis Major

The Arm Pull can be used to place the scapula into a neutral position or into an improved position while the pectoralis major is being stretched. You may be led to releasing the pectorals when no further progress can be achieved during the Arm Pull. Bring the arm in line with the horizontal fibers of the pectoralis major. Place enough traction on the arm to take up the available slack (Figure 48). Wait for the release and stretch again. Repeat until an end feel is reached.

Sometimes it will feel like the muscle does not know to relax. Maintain the traction with one hand, shifting your grip if necessary. Place your other hand on the horizontal fibers roughly in the middle of the muscle (Figure 49). Wait for the release and stretch again. Repeat until an end feel is reached.

Sometimes you will feel the release stopping at a definite point in the muscle. Maintain your traction with one hand. Place your other hand just past the restricted point and apply a countertraction. Wait for the release and stretch again. Repeat until an end feel is reached.

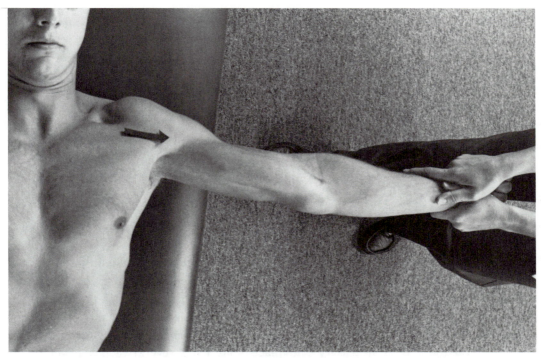

Figure 48. Stretching the horizontal fibers of the pectoralis major while performing an Arm Pull.

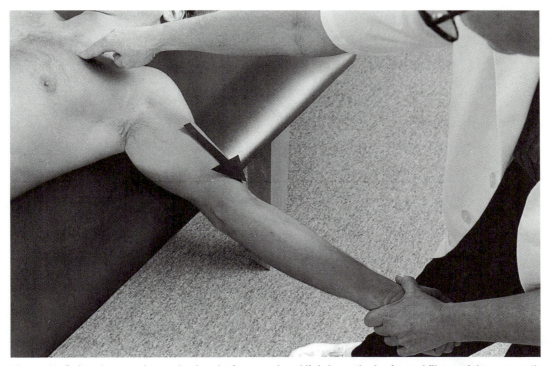

Figure 49. Cuing the muscle to relax by placing your hand lightly on the horizontal fibers of the pectoralis major.

Other times when you feel the release stopping at a definite point in the muscle, you will need to perform a trigger point release at the same time you are maintaining traction using the Arm Pull (see Trigger Point Releases on pages 123-127).

Focusing on the Diagonal Fibers of the Pectoralis Major

Bring the arm in line with the diagonal fibers of the pectoralis major. Place enough traction on the arm to take up the available slack (Figure 50). Wait for the release and stretch again. Repeat until an end feel is reached.

If it feels like the muscle does not know to relax, maintain the traction with one hand and place your other hand on the diagonal fibers with the heel of your hand roughly in the middle of the muscle. Wait for the release and stretch again. Repeat until an end feel is reached.

Focusing on the Latissimus Dorsi

With a slight change of the angle of the arm, you can change from using the Arm Pull to stretch the pectorals to stretching the latissimus dorsi. Maintain your traction on the arm with one hand while placing your other hand on the latissimus dorsi proximal to the shoulder joint (Figure 51). Apply countertraction until a release occurs and stretch again. Continue stretching that section of the muscle until no futher releases occur. Then change your grip on the arm if necessary and place your hand several inches lower on the latissimus dorsi. Apply countertraction and repeat until no further releases occur. Repeat

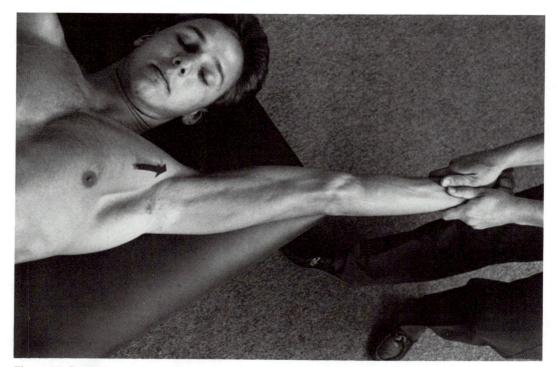

Figure 50. Stretching the lower fibers of the pectoralis major while performing an Arm Pull.

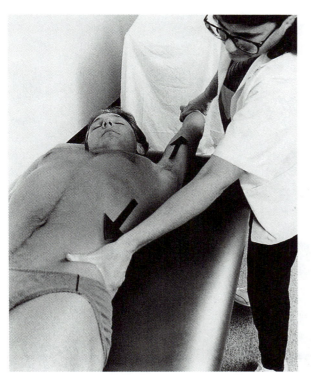

Figure 51. Stretching the latissimus dorsi with an Arm Pull while anchoring the distal attachment at the pelvis.

until you have stretched the entire latissimus dorsi in a sequential fashion. End with a full Arm Pull. Depending upon the weight of your patient, you may need to have an assistant stabilize your patient by holding him by the legs during the final Arm Pull.

Quadriceps Femoris

Stretching the quadriceps femoris requires a lot of force. Crossed hands provide you with the ability to push with the ulnar borders of your hands to apply the amount of force necessary to stretch this muscle. Be sure your hands and the patient's skin are dry before beginning this stretch to prevent your hands from slipping and pulling the leg hair.

Place your hands at the insertions of the quadriceps femoris using enough downward force to firmly anchor your hands (Figure 52). Push your hands apart until resistance is felt. Hold until a release occurs and stretch again. Repeat until an end feel is reached.

If the entire muscle will not stretch at one time, move one hand upward to the point of restriction and apply your countertraction there. Release that section of the muscle until an end feel is reached. Move your hand downward an inch or more and repeat the process, releasing the muscle sequentially until your hands are at either insertion again.

Piriformis

When the patient's major complaint is sciatica and the presence of a ruptured disc has been ruled out, stretching the piriformis will often solve this pain problem. Excess tension in this muscle can mechanically compress the sciatic nerve, no matter whether it passes over the top of the piriformis, goes through the piriformis or passes under the piriformis.

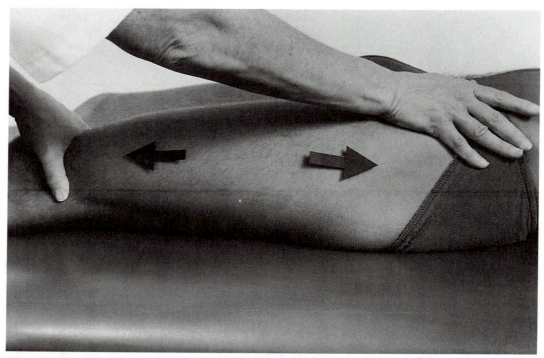

Figure 52. Stretching the quadriceps femoris.

Since the muscle cannot be palpated directly, feedback is felt through the leg which is being used as a lever.

To stretch the piriformis muscle, position your patient supine with the contralateral leg extended. The leg on the side to be stretched is flexed at the hip and knee, with the foot resting on the lateral border of the contralateral leg (Figure 53). The thigh is in internal rotation and adduction. The piriformis muscle is stretched by moving the leg into more adduction, internal rotation and hip flexion while counter pressure is applied on the barely exposed distal fibers. Wait for the release to occur and repeat until an end feel is reached.

This is one stretch your patient can easily do for himself while sitting in a chair. Instruct him to place his leg against a heavy piece of furniture and move toward it to take up the available slack. When the soft tissues relax, move closer. Repeat until an end feel is reached.

Iliopsoas

Tightness of the iliopsoas causes an increased lordotic curve, a compensating hip flexion contracture, and relative shortness and external rotation of the leg. This can be either unilateral or bilateral.[27] All of these deviations can be analyzed more readily when the patient is supine. Without adequate stabilization, compensation will substitute for true stretching. For example, if the pelvis is not prevented from rotating, hip extension may appear to be increasing when, in fact, the lordotic curve is increasing.

The iliopsoas presents a unique problem. All other muscle groups have allowed direct access to at least part of the muscle being stretched. In contrast, all portions of the iliopsoas are inaccessible to palpation. The entire technique is indirect. Using the thigh as the lever

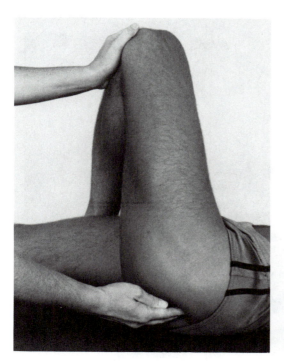

Figure 53. Stretching the piriformis with your patient supine. As the piriformis muscle relaxes, move the knee closer to the contralateral shoulder while internally rotating and adducting your patient's thigh. Pressure on the exposed fibers of the piriformis encourages relaxation through a simple feedback loop.

and the ilium as the fulcrum, the iliopsoas is stretched while keeping the pelvis in a neutral position. Feedback is transmitted through the leg and is muted by the distance it must travel.

Position your patient supine with his target buttock at or over the edge of the plinth (Figure 54). Have him flex his other hip and knee, placing his foot on the plinth. You may need to have an assistant hold him at the hip to counterbalance your stretching.

Flex his target hip to 90 degrees or more until his low back flattens and his ilium is in neutral rotation. Firmly hold the ilium in neutral with your upper hand while lowering his thigh over the edge of the plinth. Allow his thigh to abduct far enough to clear the plinth. Stop lowering his thigh when the ilium starts to rotate. Flex the hip again until the ilium is at neutral rotation.

Change your handgrip to place your other hand either on the mid-thigh or at the knee. Begin the stretch by applying traction while pushing the thigh downward (Figure 55). Wait for the release and stretch again. Because the feedback is diluted, extra care must be taken not to overpower the muscle, rather than waiting for the releases to occur.

The supine position is the position of choice if the patient has significant hip flexion contractures which prevent him from lying flat in prone. However, the iliopsoas and the other hip flexors can also be stretched with the patient prone and the hip flexed over the side of the plinth (Figure 56). This position will allow somewhat greater control over the lordotic curve because gravity will assist in holding the pelvis in a neutral position. Counterpressure is placed along the posterior rim of the pelvis, spreading the pressure out over a greater area. The major disadvantage of this position is that the therapist must support the full weight of the leg, in addition to overcoming the force of gravity while

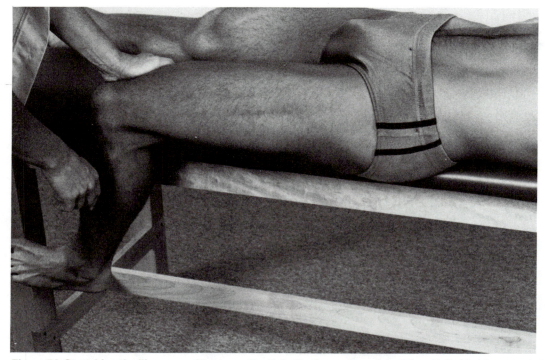

Figure 54. Stretching the iliopsoas with your patient's buttock over the edge of the plinth, his hip extended and his knee flexed.

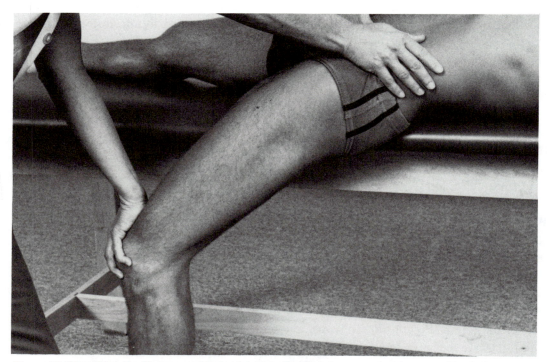

Figure 55. Stretching the iliopsoas with one hand on the ilium to prevent an increased lordotic curve and your other hand at the knee using the leg as the lever.

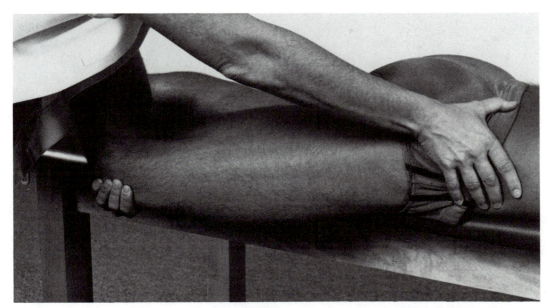

Figure 56. Stretching the iliopsoas with your patient prone and his pelvis over the edge of the plinth.

applying traction and moving the thigh into hyperextension. Again, care must be taken to wait for the releases to occur and not overpower the muscle.

If your patient is slender and has relaxed lower abdominal muscles, you may be able to place direct pressure on the lateral fibers of the psoas.[27] I have only been able to do this with female patients. Have your patient lie supine while you stand on the side of the psoas you wish to stretch. Passively flex the thigh on the pelvis with your lower hand while instructing your patient to allow her knee to flex and rest against your arm. As you flex her thigh, press your fingers along the rim of her pelvis against the lateral fibers of the psoas. Direct your fingers downward in line with the fibers of the psoas (Figure 57). Gradually lower the thigh to take up any slack in the psoas, wait for the release to occur and lower the thigh again. Continue until an end feel is reached.

Masseter

The facial muscles can be stretched using one or two hands and using one or two fingers of each hand depending upon the muscle. To prevent your hands from slipping, be sure your hands are dry and your patient's face is not oily. The masseter stretch is presented here as an example (see Figure 40). Anchor both ends of the muscle using one or two fingers of each hand. Instruct your patient to allow his jaw to remain relaxed with his teeth slightly apart. Stretch until resistance is felt. Hold until a release is felt and stretch again. Repeat until an end feel is reached. Many times it is easier to stretch a facial muscle using one hand (Figure 58) or to stretch symmetrically once you can work purely from feedback (Figure 59).

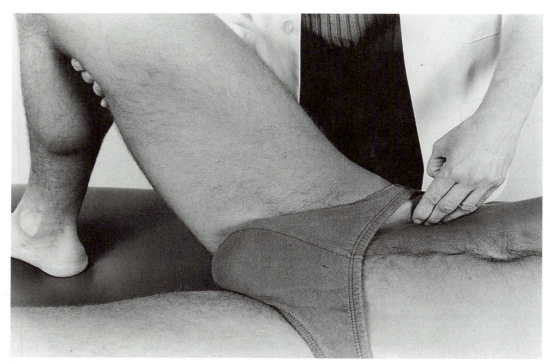

Figure 57. Directing your fingers downward along the fibers of the psoas.

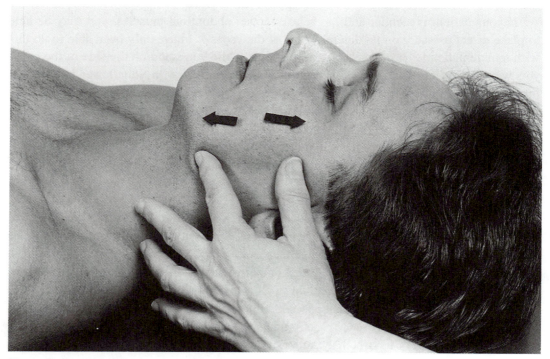

Figure 58. Stretching the masseter using one hand.

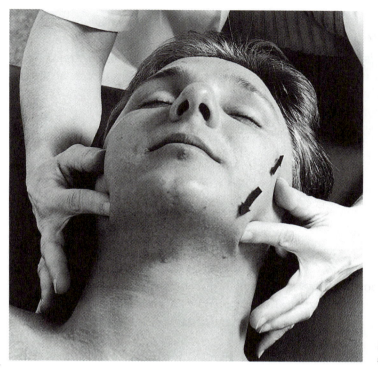

Figure 59. Symmetrical stretching of the masseter.

Sternocleidomastoid

The sternocleidomastoid has two distinct portions which must be stretched separately. Trigger points in this muscle can cause dizziness and nausea as well as radiating pain up the side of the face and into the ear. If stretching does not eliminate the trigger points, specific Trigger Point Releases must be performed. See Trigger Point Releases on pages 123-127. The sternocleidomastoid will be stretched at the same time as the posterior cervical musculature. Stretching of the posterior cervical musculature should be performed first. See pages 62-66.

Ask your patient to rotate his head to the side opposite the sternocleidomastoid you want to stretch. Place your anchoring hand at the mastoid process and your stretching hand at either the sternal or clavicular attachment. Apply enough force to take up the available slack, hold until a release occurs and stretch again. Repeat until an end feel is reached. If the entire muscle cannot be stretched, move your stretching hand to the point of restriction and stretch the muscle in sections. If the muscle cannot be stretched in sections, then specific trigger point releases must be performed. Once the trigger points are released, stretch the entire muscle at one time as described above.

Hyoid Muscles

The muscles of the anterior neck are often injured during flexion/extension injuries but are rarely treated directly. Tightness of the anterior neck muscles can cause difficulty in swallowing, speaking and jaw alignment. Before attempting these releases, explain what you propose to do to your patient and obtain **verbal consent**. You may want to review the anatomy of the anterior neck before practicing this release.

To release the suprahyoid muscles as one unit, stabilize the hyoid bone using the web space of your hand. Hook two fingers under the angle of your patient's jaw and stretch to take up the available slack. Pull the jaw upward while pushing the hyoid bone down until resistance to further stretch is felt (Figure 60). Hold until a release is felt and stretch again. Repeat until an end feel is reached. Relying on feedback, change the direction of your stretch until all of the suprahyoid muscles are released.

Change your stretching force to the base of your patient's neck and repeat for the infrahyoid muscles (Figure 61). The overlying platysma offers minimal to no resistance to this stretch.

Cervical Fascia

The prevertebral fascia continues laterally from the front of the cervical vertebrae, covering the longus colli and the scalene muscles, and extending dorsally into the fascia covering the levator scapulae muscles. Fascia extends between the muscles and attaches to the cervical vertebrae. Inferiorly, the fascia extends to the outer borders of the thorax. The space between the middle and prevertebral fascia forms the visceral compartment that houses the larynx, trachea, esophagus, thyroid gland, brachial plexus, and subclavian artery.[23, 24]

Stretching the Posterior Cervical Musculature

Position yourself comfortably at your patient's head. Cup both hands around the base of his skull and apply enough traction on the posterior cervical musculature to pull his head into capital extension by stretching the short neck extensors (Figures 62-64). Maintain traction at the base of his skull until a release is felt and then increase traction to take up the available slack. As his head is progressively pulled into capital extension, the cervical lordotic curve will decrease. If your patient's head hyperextends, ease back on your traction until his head is again in capital extension. Hold until the release occurs. You may need to change your hand position to focus attention on specific restrictions or to provide more efficient countertraction (Figure 65). Continue stretching until you reach an end feel. If your patient has difficulty relaxing in this position once you have taken up all the available slack, ease back a few degrees and ask him to inhale and exhale fully several times. Releases will often occur with exhalation.

Some patients will begin to go into spontaneous cervical movements during this release. The movements generally consist of lateral rotation and, occasionally, hyperextension and flexion of the neck. Should this occur, follow the motion, placing enough drag on his head to keep the motion slow and controlled. Spontaneous arm and leg movements feel quite different than head and neck movements. As a hesitation or restriction is felt, stop the motion until a release is achieved and then allow the motion to begin again. When a full release is achieved, the movements will stop. Your patient will relax completely, allowing you to take up slack in the muscles again. Patients who are under a lot of stress may have an emotional response to this permissive contact. When no further stretching of the posterior cervical musculature is available, have your patient take several deep breaths to be sure full relaxation has been achieved and then gently release your traction.

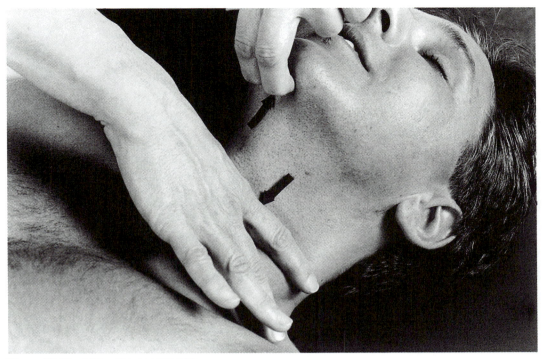

Figure 60. Stretching the suprahyoid.

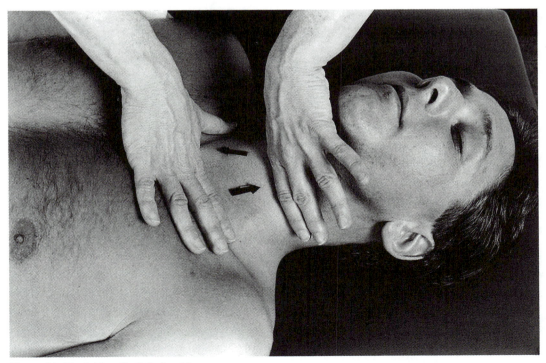

Figure 61. Stretching the infrahyoid.

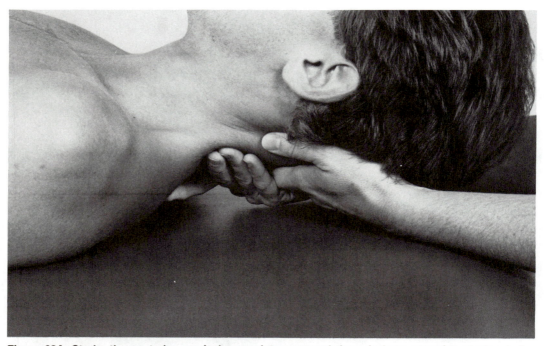

Figure 62A. Stroke the posterior cervical musculature several times in long sweeping strokes before placing both hands at the base of the occiput.

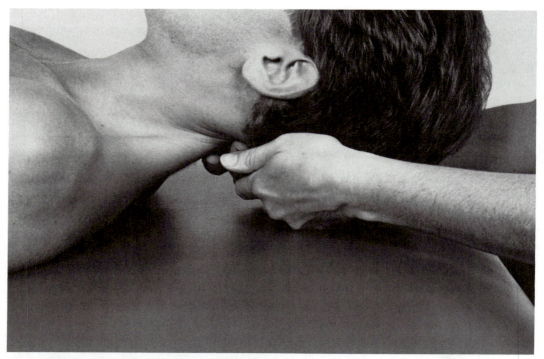

Figure 62B. As your stroking begins to relax your patient's posterior cervical musculature, you will be able to set your hands securely at the base of the occiput.

Figure 62. Beginning position for stretching of the posterior cervical musculature.

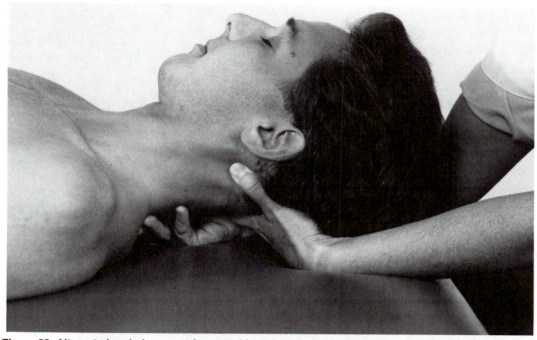

Figure 63. Alternate hand placement for stretching of the posterior cervical musculature. After stroking the posterior cervical musculature several times, place one hand at the base of the occiput and the other at the base of the neck.

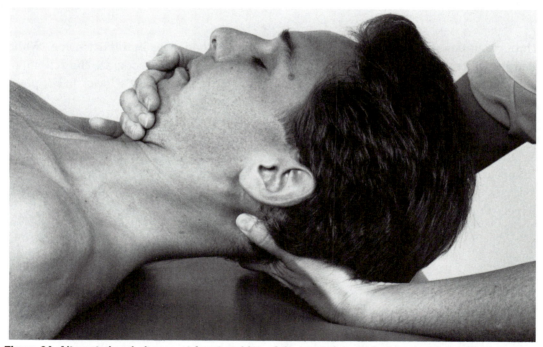

Figure 64. Alternate hand placement for stretching of the posterior cervical musculature. After stroking the posterior cervical musculature several times, place one hand at the base of the occiput and the other at the chin. With this hand placement, gentle pressure can be placed on the chin downward to counter a forward head posture. This hand placement should not be used with a patient who has temporomandibular joint (TMJ) dysfunction. Note the model's tension in the sternocleidomastoid muscle and the posterior cervical musculature.

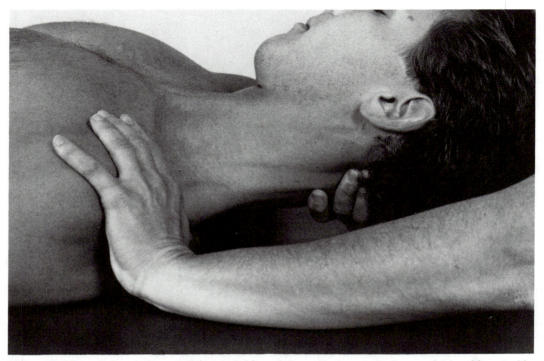

Figure 65. Alternate hand placement for stretching of the posterior cervical musculature. After stroking the posterior cervical musculature several times, place one hand at the base of the occiput and the other on the lateral neck musculature.

Throughout this release your patient should be lying with his legs in full extension. While learning this release ask your patient to cross his legs so you can recognize the sensation. If lower extremity extension causes too much stress on the patient's lower back, place pillows or a roll under his knees as you would for other treatments.

Complaints of radiating pain from active or latent myofascial trigger points at the base of the skull are common. It is impossible to avoid placing pressure on these trigger points. As the posterior cervical musculature relaxes, the radiation pattern will decrease or disappear entirely, depending on the sensitivity of the trigger points. Direct Trigger Point Releases may be necessary before maximum relaxation of these muscles is achieved. Trigger Point Releases are described on pages 123-127.

Cranial Base Release

The Cranial Base Release is often the last stretch I perform during a treatment session. This is a very tender area for most people so the initial stretch may be extremely uncomfortable. In spite of this discomfort, I have never had a patient refuse this technique. This is the time I introduce the paradox of a "good hurt" if it has not already come up. Typically, my patients will complain of significant pain and in the same breath say, "but don't stop."

When the patient's posterior cervical musculature is maximally relaxed, place the palms of your hands just under the base of his skull with your fingers extended along the

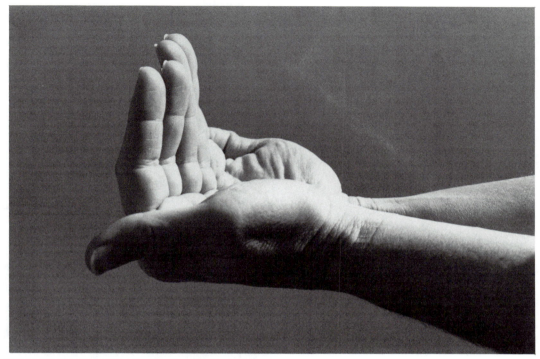

Figure 66. Hand position for the Cranial Base Release.

neck. Now flex your fingers at the metacarpal phalangeal joints so that you form a right angle to your palm with your fingertips at the base of the skull pressing firmly against the insertion of the upper trapezii (Figures 66 and 67). Instruct your patient to allow his head to drop into the palm of your hand. You may need to repeat this instruction several times because your patient will have the tendency to try to hold his head up off your fingertips. As progressive relaxation of the muscles occurs, slide the back of your hands slightly more toward your patient's feet while angling your fingers toward the top of his head and applying an upward traction force. This allows you to hook your fingers under the base of the skull and put inhibitory pressure on the deeper muscles while maintaining your upward traction. Your patient's head will slowly drop into your hands and stretch upward toward you (Figure 68). As the short neck extensors relax and stretch, your patient's chin will tuck.

Your hand and finger strength will determine how you want to finish this particular stretch. The first method is to continue cradling the skull in the palms of your hands and maintain traction with your second and third fingers, while placing your fourth finger on the patient's first and second cervical vertebrae. Extend the fourth finger to distract the vertebrae while flexing the second and third fingers to traction the skull gently from the upper cervical spine (Figure 69). When no further movement occurs, again place traction on the posterior cervical musculature, moving into the last few degrees of capital extension (Figure 70).

The second method is to continue maintaining traction upward with your palms and extend your fingers along your patient's neck and the base of the skull. Apply forceful

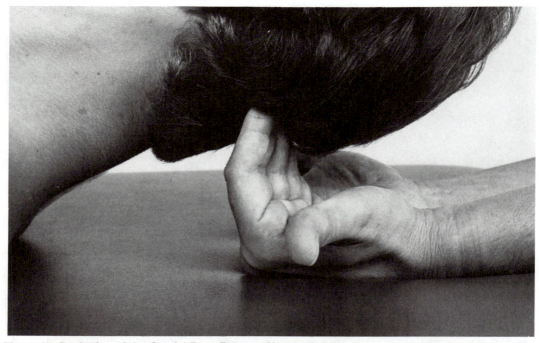

Figure 67. Beginning of the Cranial Base Release. Your patient's head rests on your fingertips placing pressure on the proximal fibers of the posterior cervical musculature. Very often this is the site of active myofascial trigger points that cause radiating pain into the head. Some patients are initially unable to tolerate enough pressure to allow the cranial base to release. Others will talk of a good hurt and welcome the pressure.

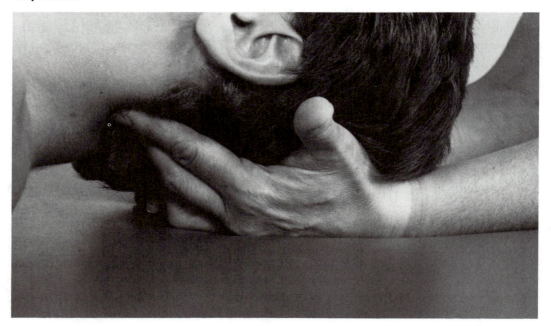

Figure 68. End of the Cranial Base Release. Your patient's head rests in your palms as his skull is being distracted from the upper cervical vertebrae.

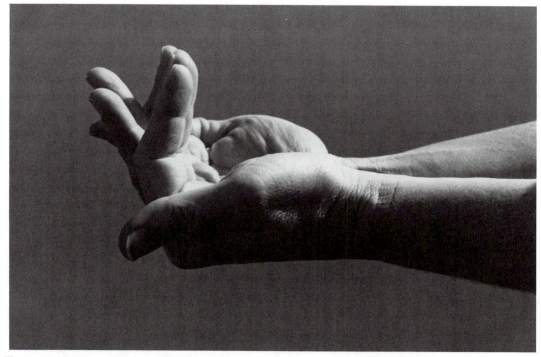

Figure 69. Hand position for distracting the skull from the upper cervical vertebrae.

traction by rocking your upper body backward while maintaining your grip (Figure 71). Hold until you feel the head become heavy and the muscles become soft.

This is a very sensitive area where myofascial trigger points, either active or latent, may be present. In the process of performing this release, digital pressure is placed on these trigger points and may release them as well. If these trigger points are so sensitive that your patient is unable to tolerate the amount of pressure needed to complete the release, several treatment sessions to treat the trigger points may be necessary before the cranial base is finally released.

The base of the skull is a prime area for injury during a flexion/extension injury. This common injury results in the activation of multiple trigger points at the base of the skull, throughout the posterior cervical musculature and the sternocleidomastoid muscles. All of these trigger points may need to be returned to latent status before a Cranial Base Release is successful.

Spontaneous movement of the head and neck may occur during a Cranial Base Release, reproducing the motions that resulted in the original myofascial injury. Continue to follow the motion, placing enough drag on the movement to keep it slow and controlled until your patient finally relaxes and permits the Cranial Base Release to be completed. An emotional response may also be triggered in this position.[16]

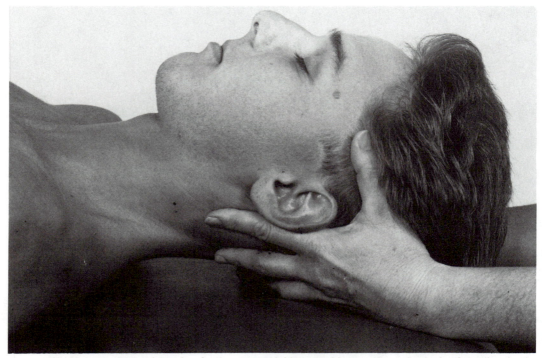

Figure 70A. Note the lack of tension in the sternocleidomastoid as well as the lack of tension in the posterior cervical musculature.

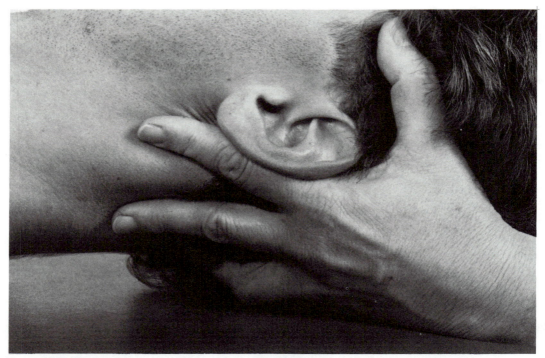

Figure 70B. The head is in complete contact with the therapist's hands and the cervical lordosis is flattened. Note the distance between the neck and the plinth. Compare with Figure 68.

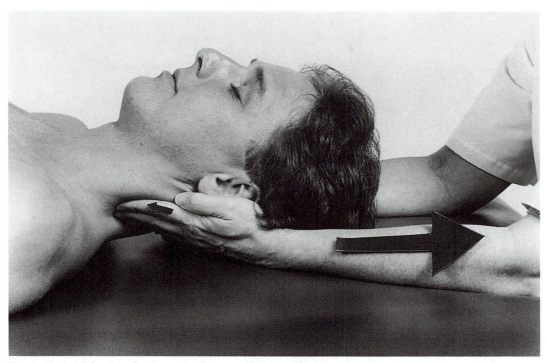

Figure 71. Applying traction by extending your fingers along the neck with the heel of your hand against the cranial base.

Thoracic Inlet Release

Before performing a Thoracic Inlet Release, you must explain the purpose of this release to your patient and be sure both of you have a clear understanding of the need for this release. When working with a woman, you must be clear there is no sexual intent although your hand may contact her breast tissue. If your patient expresses any reluctance or uneasiness with this release, do not proceed until you have been given specific consent.

This is never the first release I use. Usually, I will have begun treating the posterior cervical musculature which naturally leads me to the tightness in the anterior chest wall. By this time my patient has a good idea of her response to Myofascial Release and will be comfortable with my hand on her anterior chest wall.

If you have already stretched the posterior cervical musculature, the best position from which to perform this release is sitting at the patient's head (Figure 72). If you intend to stretch other muscles in the trunk or to perform an Arm Pull next, this maneuver can be performed sitting at the patient's side (Figure 73).

Sitting at your patient's head, place your non-dominant hand under the patient's lower cervical region and upper thoracic spine (Figure 74). Place your dominant hand at the midline of the chest just below the sternal notch (Figure 75). This will place your forearm and elbow along the patient's cheek. Most often this is a very comfortable position, both for the therapist and the patient, allowing maximum contact and relaxation. This also transmits a sensation of security to your patient, and you may feel a progressive relaxation

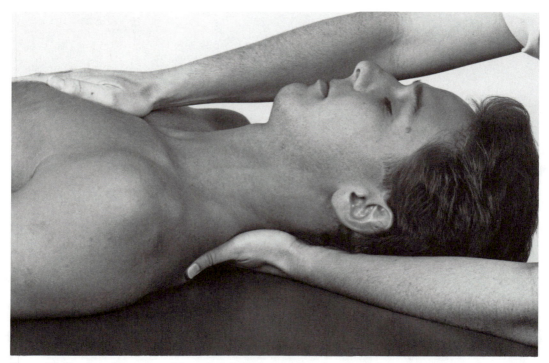

Figure 72. Hand positions for a Thoracic Inlet Release when the cervical musculature is to be stretched next.

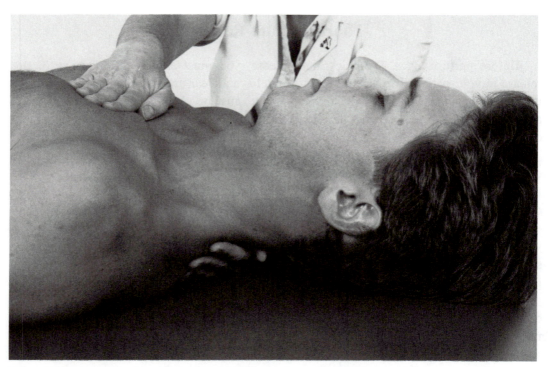

Figure 73. Side position for a Thoracic Inlet Release when other horizontal releases are to be performed next.

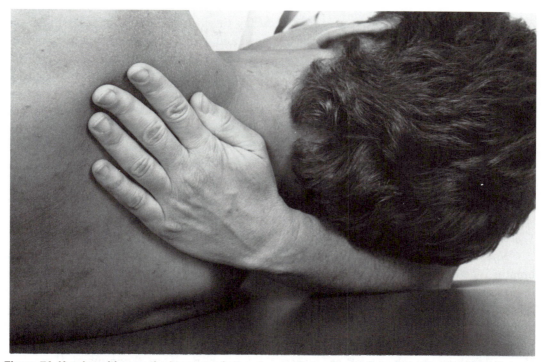

Figure 74. Hand position on the lower cervical and upper thoracic vertebrae for a Thoracic Inlet Release performed from the side position.

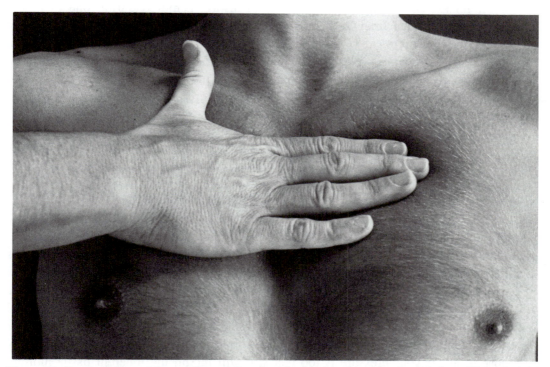

Figure 75. Hand position at the midline of the chest just below the sternal notch for a Thoracic Inlet Release performed from the side position.

of the head and neck against your forearm during this release. Once again, instruct your patient to lie with both lower extremities extended and without crossing her legs or ankles.

Your pressure on the chest should be fairly light to prevent direct inhibition of the inherent tissue motion. Compress your patient's body between your hands until a resistance is felt. Lighten your pressure until you begin to feel the inherent tissue motion. This is the proper amount of pressure to use. When first learning to perform the horizontal releases, you may want to ask your patient to give you feedback on the amount of pressure you are using until you are able to utilize the feedback from your hands. Once you have learned the technique, you may find you are using a heavier touch than when you started.

The inherent tissue motion will guide your hand in a roughly circular or oval pattern across the chest wall. At an area of restriction, the motion will cease. Keep your hand in the same position with the same amount of pressure pushing against the restriction and wait. When a release is achieved, the inherent tissue motion will resume.

When no further releases are possible, your patient may signal by taking a deep sighing breath. Whether this occurs or not, you will feel a softening throughout the entire thoracic region and a profound relaxation when the end point is reached. At this point, no further relaxation is available. It is very easy to override your patient's inherent tissue motion by using too much pressure. If this happens, lighten your touch until you feel the movement resume. The easiest way to lighten your touch is to think to yourself, "lighter, lighter." You will feel your touch ease off as you respond to your own internal command. If you lose the feel of the movement by losing your concentration, clear your mind of distractions and refocus your attention to the sensations under your hands.

A full release of the thoracic region is not always achieved during one treatment session. If the Thoracic Inlet Release is being used as preparation for other stretching maneuvers, the procedure can be terminated after a partial release of the tension. However, if your goal of treatment is relaxation of the chest wall, specific stretching of the more superficial tense muscles, such as the pectoralis major, may be needed before the anterior chest wall can be fully relaxed. Trust what you feel under your hands to direct you to the next tense area to be relaxed.

Diaphragm Release

The Diaphragm Release is performed in the same manner as the Thoracic Inlet Release. For this release, sit at the patient's side, perpendicular to the line of the diaphragm. Place your dominant hand on the patient's abdomen at the base of the rib cage (Figure 76), and your non-dominant hand posteriorly over the diaphragm (Figure 77). Press your hands together with firm pressure until resistance stops further inward movement of your hands. Relax the tension in your arms and shoulders to lighten your pressure. Sit quietly until you feel your patient's inherent tissue motion drawing your upper hand in a circular or oval fashion, across the lower rib cage and abdominal wall. At the same time you may feel your lower hand being drawn in a reverse pattern from your other hand or your lower hand may not move at all. If your pressure is too heavy, it will inhibit the inherent tissue motion. Therefore, if movement has not started within 30 seconds, lighten your pressure again until you begin to feel the inherent tissue motion begin.

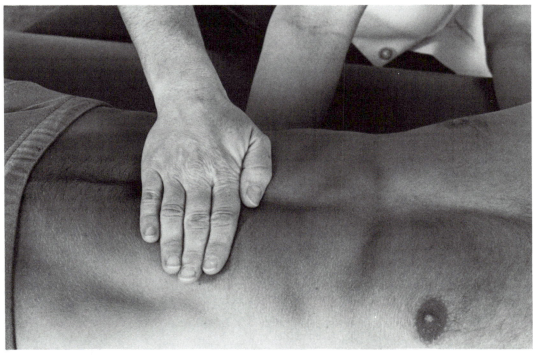

Figure 76. Hand position on the upper abdomen for the Diaphragm Release.

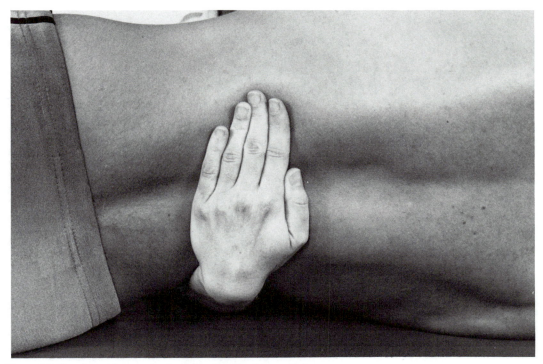

Figure 77. Hand position on the back for the Diaphragm Release.

Follow this movement without attempting to direct it. When or if you begin to retrace the same path several times, begin to add a slight additional pressure along the tightest borders of the pattern. As you add additional pressure outward to enlarge the movement, your hand may be drawn in a different direction as tension is released in a three-dimensional manner throughout the abdomen. Continue to follow the inherent tissue motion until no further movement is present or you are led to a different area of the body.

Pelvic Floor Release

The Pelvic Floor Release is performed in the same manner as the Thoracic Inlet and Diaphragm Releases. Be sure your patient has an empty bladder before beginning this release. Place your non-dominant hand under the patient's coccyx (Figure 78) and your dominant hand just above his pubis symphysis (Figure 79). Compress the lower abdomen between your hands until resistance to further compression is felt. Allow your touch to lighten until you feel the inherent tissue motion begin to lead your hand around the lower abdomen. Follow the motion, releasing restrictions as described above until no further restrictions are felt. Often an anterior-posterior rocking of the pelvis is felt when the release is achieved. This should be smooth, rhythmic and symmetrical in nature. Feeling this movement is a signal that full release has been achieved.

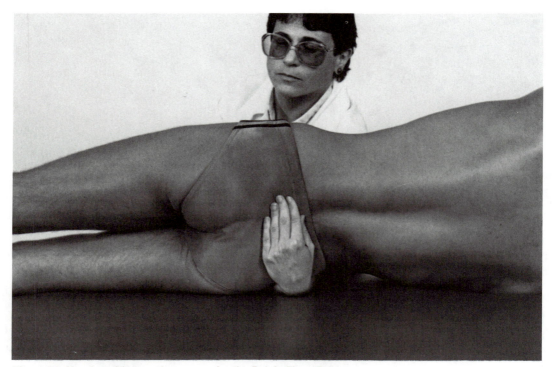

Figure 78. Hand position on the coccyx for the Pelvic Floor Release.

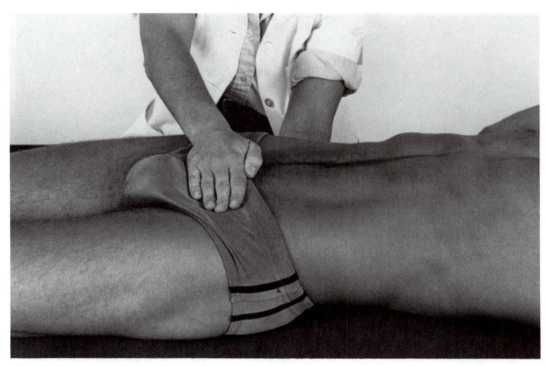

Figure 79. Hand position on the lower abdomen just above the pubis symphysis for the Pelvic Floor Release.

If your patient has endometriosis or scarring from a surgical procedure, she may complain of a "good" stretch pain as adhesions are stretched and/or broken. This release can sometimes relieve menstrual cramps.

Bilateral Arm Pull

Depending upon what other structures you want to stretch, position your patient supine (Figure 80) or prone (Figure 81) with his arms extended overhead. Grasp both of your patient's wrists with your hands. Place traction on both arms as evenly as possible, keeping the arms adducted to the head and taking up the available slack. Hold this position until the soft tissues relax. Increase your traction slightly, taking up the additional slack. Repeat this process until no further stretch is possible and an end feel is reached. Slowly begin to abduct both arms to determine if further tightness is present and can be released. When no further tightness is present, gently release your traction and return your patient's arms to his sides.

Shoulder flexion with the patient supine will focus the stretch of the shoulder girdles on the pectoral muscles, the latissimus dorsi and the entire upper thoracic region. In contrast, the same stretch with the patient prone will focus stretch on the erector spinae muscles and the parascapular muscles as well as the entire upper thoracic region.

If spontaneous arm movements begin, maintain traction and place drag on both arms to keep the movements slow and controlled. When hesitations or skips occur, stop the

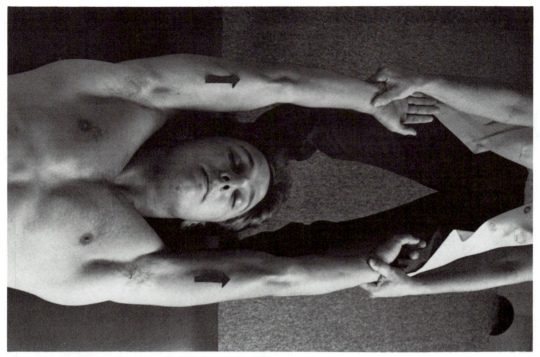

Figure 80. Supine position for the Bilateral Arm Pull.

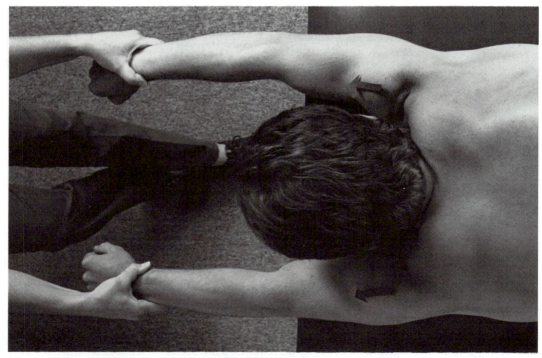

Figure 81. Prone position for the Bilateral Arm Pull.

movement, hold until a release occurs and take up the slack as described above. If one arm moves more rapidly than the other, you may need to let go of the less active arm and follow the motion of the more active arm. Once that arm is quiet, resume symmetrical traction and follow the motion of the other arm. When both arms are quiet, resume symmetrical traction again. Repeat until an end feel is reached.

Bilateral Leg Pull

Instruct your patient to "lie heavily" on the plinth. With your patient supine, cup both heels in your hands and apply enough traction to take up the available slack (Figure 82). Maintain a steady traction until a release occurs and then increase your traction to take up the additional slack. Repeat until no further stretch is possible and an end feel is reached. If spontaneous movement of the legs begins, maintain your traction and place enough drag on the legs to keep the movement slow. If you feel any skips or hesitations, stop the motion. Move the legs back a few degrees and hold until the release occurs. Allow the movement to resume. Continue until an end feel is reached. If one leg is moving more than the other, you may need to release the quieter leg and follow the movement of the more active one until an end feel is reached. Then return to the Bilateral Leg Pull until an end feel is present in both legs.

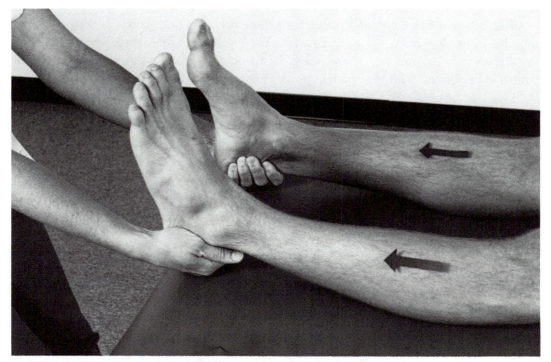

Figure 82. Hand position for the Bilateral Leg Pull with the patient supine.

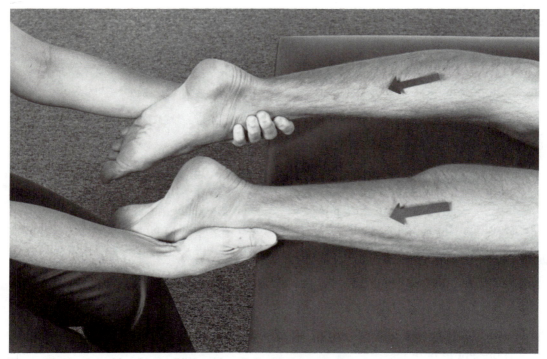

Figure 83. Hand position for the Bilateral Leg Pull with the patient prone.

The Bilateral Leg Pull allows stretching to be achieved throughout the erector spinae muscles in the low back, the quadratus laborum muscles and the lower abdominals. The hip flexors can be stretched if the pelvis is maintained in a neutral position when this stretch is performed with your patient prone (Figure 83).

Superficial Skin Releases

Immobility of the skin is the most superficial restriction to free movement. Often these restrictions are eliminated during other techniques. However, superficial skin restrictions must be specifically addressed when they impede your ability to feel and treat deeper restrictions. Depending on the body part being tested, either the palm or the fingertips is used to detect restrictions. On broad body surfaces, the palm is placed firmly on the skin with enough force to maintain contact while the skin is moved upward, downward and from side to side to feel for free movement (Figures 84-87). This testing procedure may release some superficial restrictions. When restrictions are found, Skin Rolling or J Stroking will usually release them quickly.

Skin Rolling
A very easy method of releasing superficial restrictions is Skin Rolling. In an area with minimal or no restrictions, the skin can be smoothly rolled between the thumb and fingers of the therapist. Any restrictions will release quickly and smoothly with very little effort.

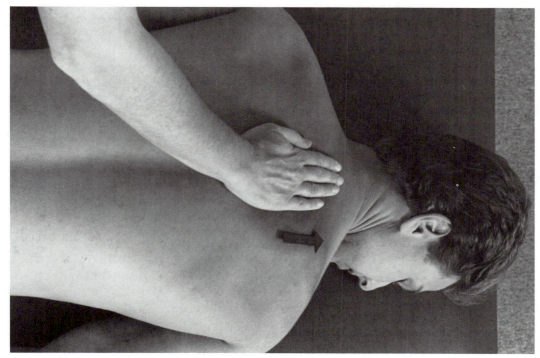

Figure 84A. Upward.

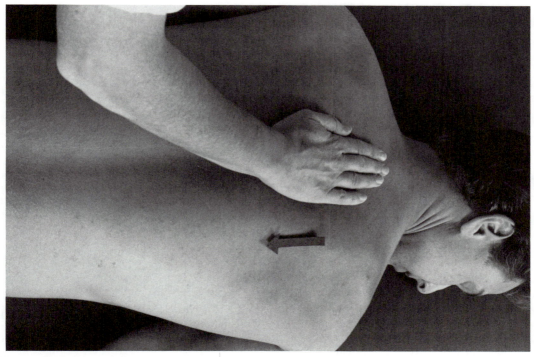

Figure 84B. Downward.

Figure 84. Testing for thoracic skin mobility. No restriction of movement is demonstrated in this series of illustrations.

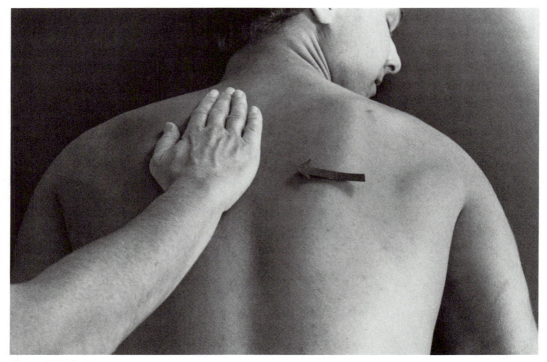

Figure 84C. Left.

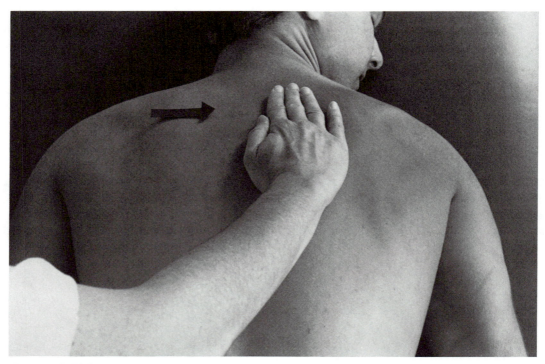

Figure 84D. Right.

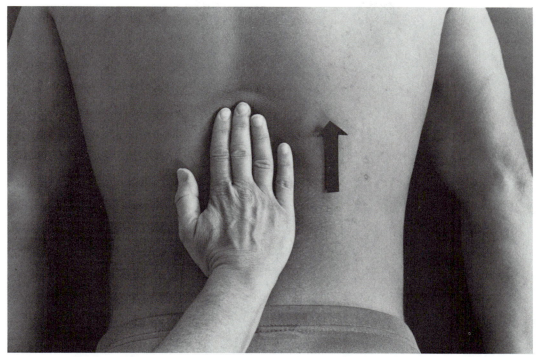

Figure 85A. Upward mobility is restricted. Note the bunching of the skin in front of the therapist's fingers.

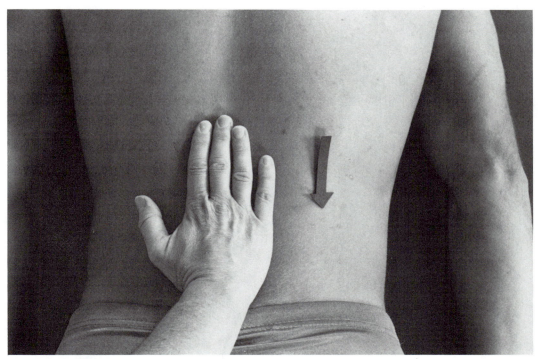

Figure 85B. Downward.

Figure 85. Testing for low back skin mobility.

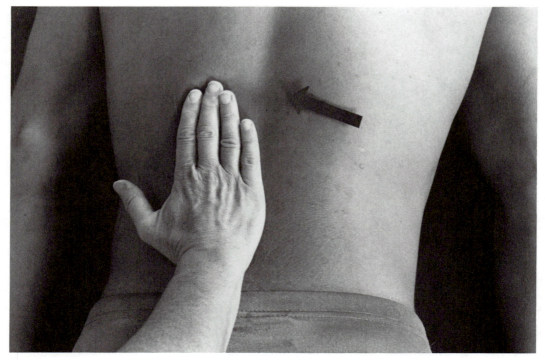

Figure 85C. Left.

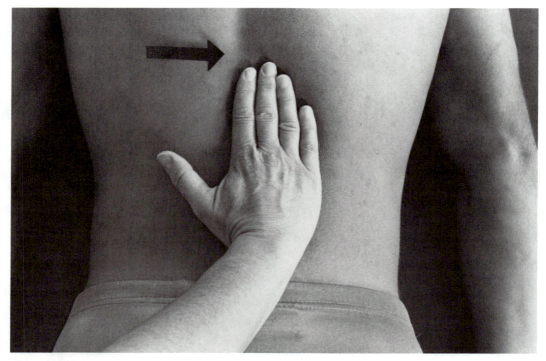

Figure 85D. Right.

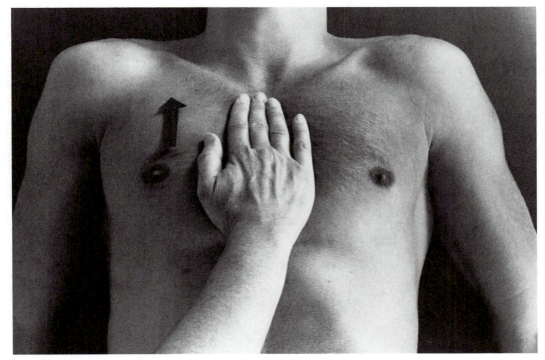

Figure 86A. Upward.

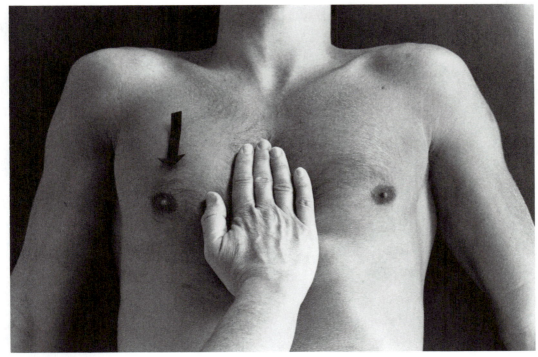

Figure 86B. Downward.

Figure 86. Testing for anterior chest wall skin mobility. No restriction of movement is demonstrated.

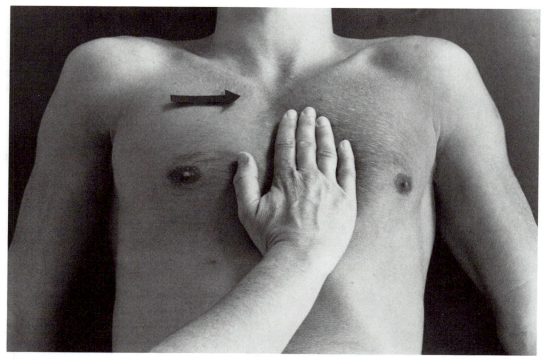

Figure 86C. Left.

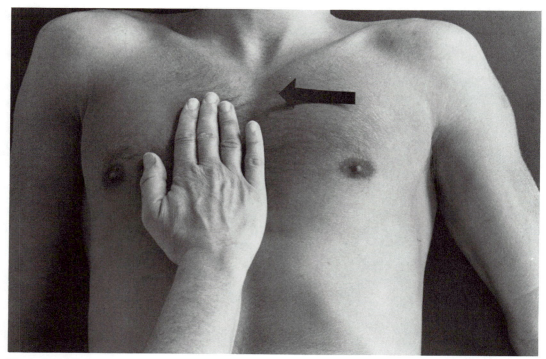

Figure 86D. Right.

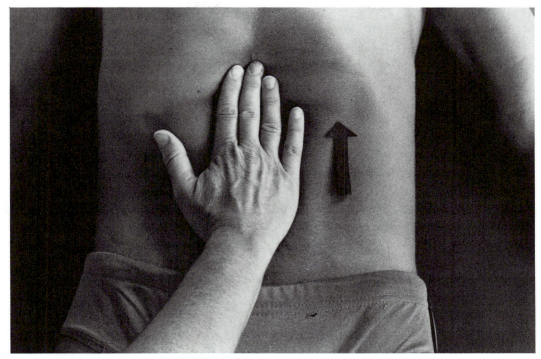

Figure 87A. Upward.

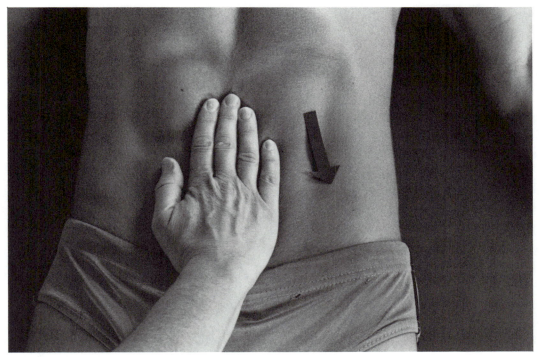

Figure 87B. Downward.

Figure 87. Testing for abdominal skin mobility.

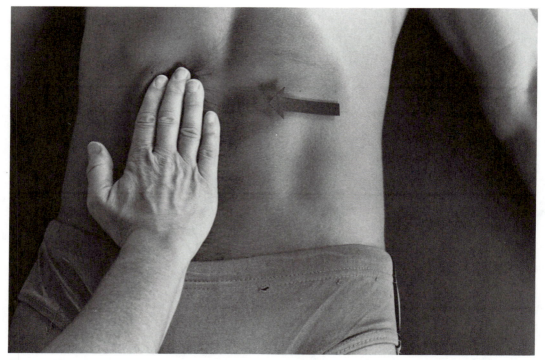

Figure 87C. Left. Note the restriction of movement and the bunching of the skin next to the therapist's hand.

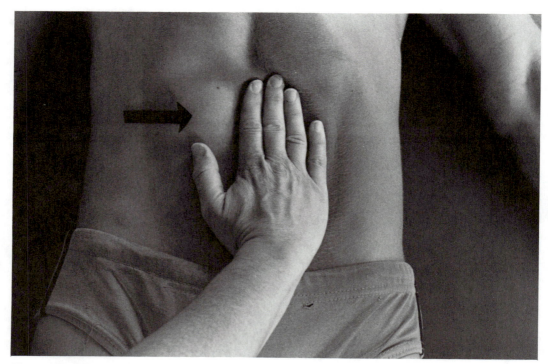

Figure 87D. Right.

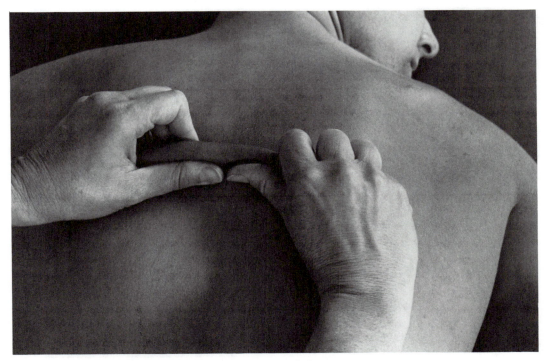

Figure 88. Skin Rolling for the release of superficial restrictions.

When stronger restrictions are felt, use slightly greater force to lift the skin upward to take up the available slack. Wait for the release to occur and then roll the skin slightly forward, repeating the same process until all restrictions are released. In some instances it will be necessary to repeat this movement, taking the skin both forward and backward until all restrictions to free skin movement are released (Figure 88).

This same technique can be used to release scar tissue when enough skin area is available in which to work, such as in the abdominal or thoracic regions (Figure 89). Trigger points which are located in the skin will be quickly released with skin rolling.

J Stroking

If it is not possible to use Skin Rolling or if Skin Rolling is not adequate, J Stroking can be used across restrictions. This technique does not rely on feedback from the patient, but is done with specific restrictions in mind. The J Stroking procedure is similar to connective tissue massage with definite lines of stroking to be followed.[28] However, when used with Myofascial Release, J Stroking is performed only in an area identified in the assessment as restricted, and not throughout a generalized area.

To perform a J Stroke release, use firm contact to stretch the skin to take up the slack (Figure 90). With the second and third fingers held against each other for added strength and stability, firmly draw short J's on the patient's skin, progressively moving across the restricted area. The hook part of the J should be drawn across the restriction while the straight part goes along the same line as the restriction. Reassess the area by again moving the skin in all directions with your hand flat. If all restrictions are not released, repeat J Stroking, moving at a 45 degree angle from your first J's. Repeat until all restrictions are released.

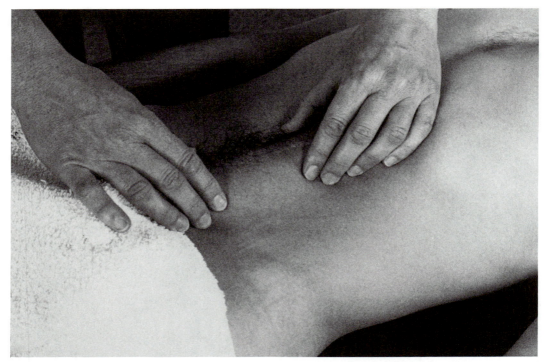

Figure 89. Releasing scar tissue. The scar is gathered in a pincer grip and lifted upward from the body. As adhesions release, the scar is distracted farther from the body.

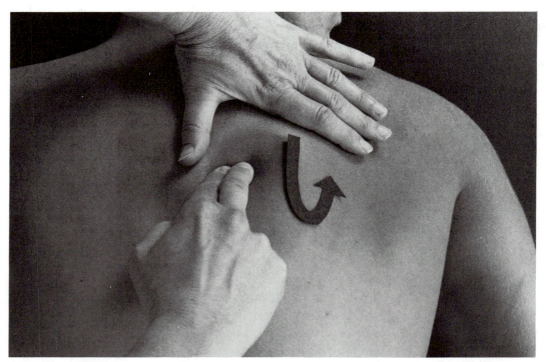

Figure 90. Hand placement for J Stroking. The upper hand must stretch and stabilize the skin above the area of restriction to eliminate extraneous movement which would prevent stretching of the restrictions.

Transient hyperemia may be present following this treatment. In addition, your patient may complain of a burning or tearing sensation during or immediately after this technique.[29] This is a normal response to a release of adhesions and does not indicate fresh injury to the tissues. This burning or tearing sensation usual disappears quickly but may last several hours in very sensitive people.

III

Advanced Techniques

Introduction to Advanced Techniques

As you refine your skill of responding to feedback from your patient's body, you gradually move into more advanced treatment techniques, responding to very subtle changes which you would not have noticed before. Sometimes you surprise yourself, not quite knowing why your hands are moving the way they are. In addition, you are able to feel differences in muscle tension depending upon the abduction or adduction of your patient's extremities. When an assistant is available, you can direct how you want the patient moved to facilitate a release of tension (Figure 91), and you can feel the change in tension when the patient actively moves.

You can find the restrictions in the upper part of your patient's body by simply placing your hand(s) on his posterior cervical musculature. Soon you will be able to sense the restrictions throughout his body from any "listening point" (Figure 92) and decide which restriction should be treated first.

Fine tuning of stretch is easier with multi-person techniques. With your patient either supine or prone on the plinth, a target myofascial unit can be stretched in two and sometimes three dimensions at the same time. You must be able to direct your assistants to move the patient's body to positions of greatest ease. Just by placing your patient's body in these positions, you will feel releases occuring as the body responds to this temporary proper alignment. Still, for a total stretch you must learn to treat in three dimensions, working with your patient seated or standing. Treatment in three dimensions is done entirely on feedback and requires the highest of skills.

There are a few additional single person techniques which cannot be learned until you reach this level of expertise and sensitivity. The Hair Pull is used to release scalp restrictions and can be the finishing stretch for the Cranial Base Release. The Ear Pull relieves tension in the jaw and around the temporomandibular joints. Trigger Point Releases must be learned in isolation before combining them with Focused Stretching. Releasing the Dural Tube is performed entirely on feedback.

You have felt your patient's spontaneous movement and now you are ready to facilitate that movement as you use your hands to place your patient in a light hypnotic trance.[15,29] As you match your patient's movements and rhythms, you will notice a new smoothness of movement and an ability to focus so completely on your patient that neither of you can be distracted.

Hair Pull

The Hair Pull is a Superficial Skin Release which can affect the tension throughout the scalp, face and anterior neck. It can be used to indirectly approach facial and jaw restrictions which the patient cannot let you treat in a more direct manner. Once again, very clear boundaries are essential to prevent your patient from misunderstanding what you are doing. Hair pulling is a uniquely female mode of fighting and abuse. Abuse memories can be activated and can trigger an emotional release.[15,16] If this happens, I encourage my patient to express her feelings in whatever manner works for her.

When preparing to perform the Hair Pull, have your patient move down on the plinth to allow you to have your arm fully supported. If your arm or hand slips, you will sharply pull your patient's hair, triggering reflex muscle contraction and causing unnecessary pain.

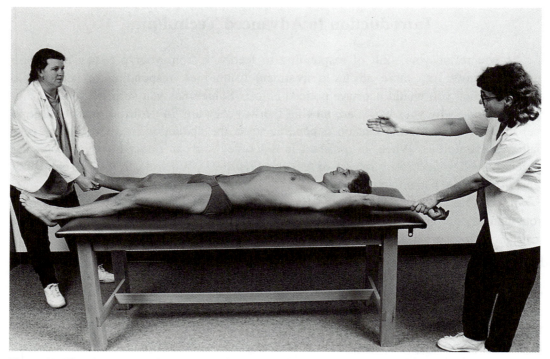

Figure 91. Directing your assistant to passively move the patient's leg to facilitate a release of tension.

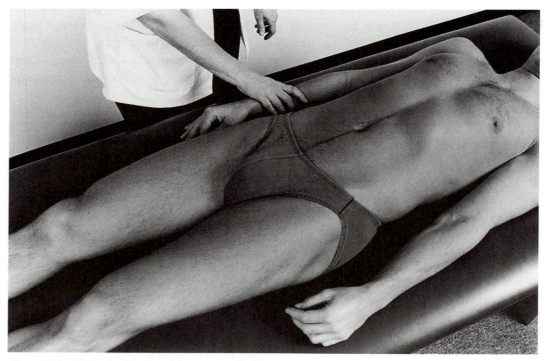

Figure 92A. "Listening" by touching your patient's arm.

Figure 92. Changes in the inherent tissue motion can be detected by "listening" with your hands from any part of your patient's body.

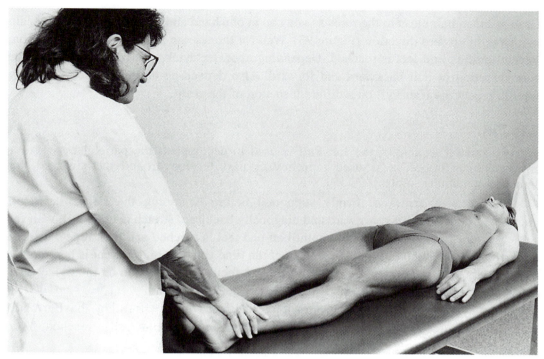

Figure 92B. "Listening" by holding your patient's legs.

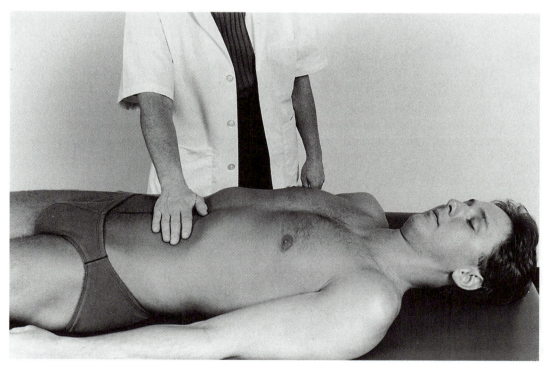

Figure 92C. "Listening" by placing your hand on your patient's abdomen.

Grab as much hair close to the roots as you can in one hand and begin to traction the scalp in a straight upward direction (Figure 93). Wait for the release and increase your traction. Repeat until an end feel is reached. Depending upon feedback, you may want to change your direction of pull backward and forward. Also depending upon feedback, you may want to repeat the Hair Pull on a different section of the scalp.

Ear Pull

As a cranial technique, the Ear Pull is used to decompress the parietal bone. As a myofascial technique, it is used to relieve excess tension around the jaw and the temporomandibular joints.

Be sure your arms are firmly supported before beginning the Ear Pull. Begin tractioning both ears in a downward and diagonally backward stretch (Figure 94). Wait for a release and stretch again. Continue until an end feel is reached and then repeat using a straight backward stretch (Figure 95). Most of the time you will find one ear is less mobile than the other. Maintain traction on both ears, but focus your attention on the tighter side until both are equally mobile or an end feel is reached.

You may feel spontaneous movement of the jaw when performing the Ear Pull. Maintain your traction to place drag on the motion until an end feel is reached. Your patient may feel releases occurring throughout her face, mouth and throat.

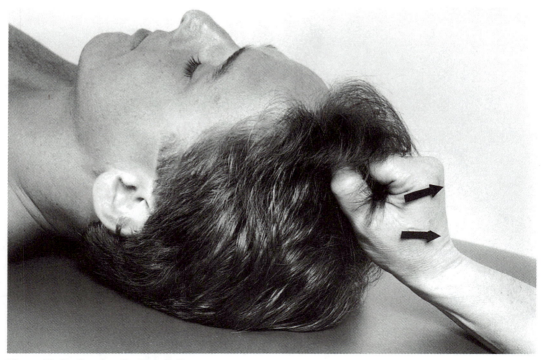

Figure 93. Performing the Hair Pull.

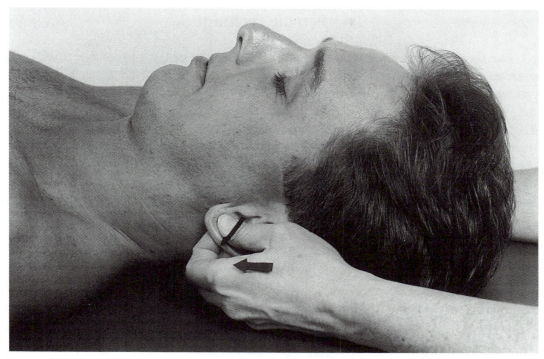

Figure 94. Performing the Ear Pull tractioning diagonally and downward.

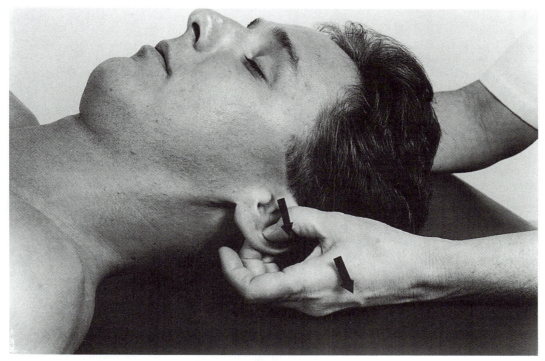

Figure 95. Performing the Ear Pull tractioning straight backward.

Two Person Techniques

Two therapists can more efficiently stretch large areas of the body at one time. Long muscles like the latissimus dorsi are difficult to stretch because all of its attachments cannot be anchored at the same time using a single person technique. Other muscles like the pectorals can be more efficiently stretched when a simultaneous Arm Pull is performed. The Arm Pull takes up the available slack in the pectorals and puts the muscle fibers in their end range, allowing Focused Stretching to proceed more quickly.

Most therapists do not have the luxury of having another therapist to assist them when using Myofascial Release. I have on occasion asked my office manager or my secretary to assist me in performing these stretches. Once you have developed the sensitivity of your hands, you will be able to direct your assistant to perform the complementary stretch to what you are doing.

Bilateral Straight Arm and Leg Pull–Symmetrical Stretch

Two people can perform simultaneous Arm and Leg Pulls with the patient either supine or prone (Figures 96 and 97). Each must counterbalance the other's pull to avoid dragging the patient in either direction. If this traction is applied in a timid fashion, no true stretching will occur. Spontaneous mobilization of the vertebrae, costovertebral and costrosternal joints may occur during this stretch.

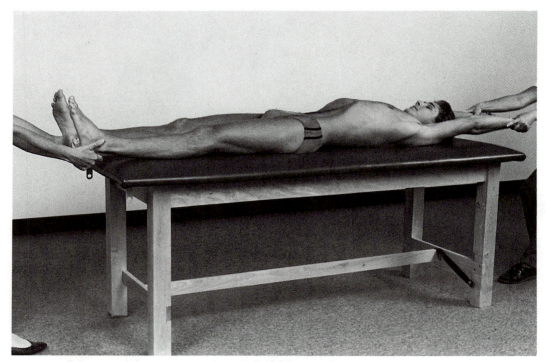

Figure 96. Two person Bilateral Arm and Leg Pull with your patient supine.

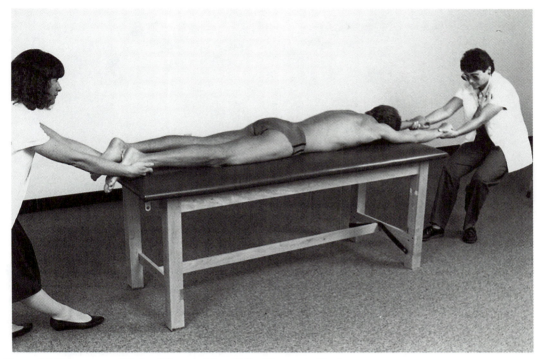

Figure 97. Two person Bilateral Arm and Leg Pull with your patient prone.

Instruct your assistant to begin applying traction gradually as you counterbalance with your own traction. When no further stretch is available, hold until the release is felt and increase your traction. Repeat until an end feel is reached. If no further stretch is possible, but an end feel is not reached, stop this stretch and perform a focused stretch of the restricted area. Once that is released, resume the symmetrical stretch.

Bilateral Curved Arm and Leg Pull–Symmetrical Stretch

Stretching into a convex/concave position can be used to place the targeted vertebrae in an open position and to stretch the small muscles between those vertebrae (Figures 98 and 99). This position also allows for spontaneous mobilization of the facet joints on the convex side.

After instructing your patient to "lie heavily" on the table and not move his hips, have your assistant begin applying traction gradually as you counterbalance with your own traction. When no further stretch is available, change your angle of pull to move your patient into a concave position (see Figures 98 and 99). Hold until the release occurs and increase your traction to stretch again. Repeat until an end feel is reached. Return to your original straight stretch, hold until a release occurs and stretch again. If no release occurs, move your patient into the opposite concave position. Hold until the release occurs and increase your traction to stretch again. Repeat until an end feel is reached. Return to the straight symmetrical position to finish this stretch.

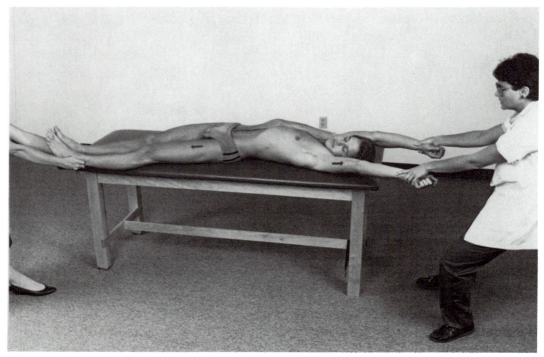

Figure 98. Two person Bilateral Concave Arm and Leg Pull with your patient supine.

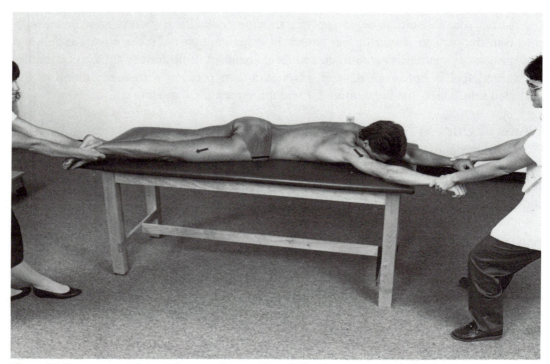

Figure 99. Two person Bilateral Concave Arm and Leg Pull with your patient prone.

Ipsilateral Arm and Leg Pull–Symmetrical Stretch

Once the Bilateral Symmetrical Stretch is completed, further stretch can be achieved using the patient's arm and leg on the same side to release unilateral tightness. Tractioning the arm and leg on the same side of the body is an effective way to stretch the latissimus dorsi, the quadratus lumborum and the intercostal muscles. This can be a more efficient approach to stretching these muscles than attempting to stretch them directly.

This stretch can be performed with the patient prone, supine or side-lying depending upon the target muscle (Figure 100). Multiple variations of side-lying can be used to further isolate the target muscle.

Contralateral Arm and Leg Pull–Asymmetrical Stretch

A contralateral stretch effectively releases restrictions which cross the midline of the body. There is no anatomic structure which crosses the midline other than the fascia. Your patient can be either prone or supine for this stretch depending upon which myofascial groups you wish to target. A prone position can be used to focus on the iliopsoas, the trapezii, and the serratus anterior (Figure 101). The supine position can be used to focus on the obliques, the pectorals, the iliopsoas and the intercostals (Figure 102).

Visualize the line of stretch going from one arm to the contralateral leg and running through the external oblique on one side and the internal oblique on the other. Use this line as your starting position unless your hands tell you otherwise. With the therapist at the patient's head acting as leader, begin to traction the arm and leg evenly. As restrictions are felt, pause, wait for the release to occur, then increase your traction to take up the available slack. Repeat until an end feel is reached.

A restriction can encompass all fibers in a muscle or a subset of them. If the only restrictions present include all muscle fibers in the target muscle, most often the releases will occur in a smooth sequential manner when the arm and leg are lined up. If there is uneven tightness in the target muscle, the releases will feel jerky or ratchety. You may need to make small adjustments in the position of the arm and leg as each release occurs.

Change the angle of the arm or the leg or both to place each restriction in a position of greatest ease. As one restriction releases, you will need to change your angle of pull to place the next one in a position of greatest ease. Once the lead therapist feels no further restrictions, the other therapist may still detect tightness in the lower part of the patient's body. If that happens, switch roles so the other therapist can direct body position to release recalcitrant restrictions in the lower half of the patient's body. If your assistant is not accomplished in Myofascial Release, switch positions with your assistant to continue stretching your patient's lower body. Do not neglect your patient's verbal feedback during this stretch. Your patient may be able to direct you to restrictions your hands are not yet sensitive enough to detect.

When you can detect no further restrictions, repeat your original diagonal stretch and then switch to the patient's opposite arm and leg. When both diagonals are fully stretched, repeat the Symmetrical Arm and Leg Pulls for final symmetrical stretching. Always finish a treatment session with a symmetrical stretch.

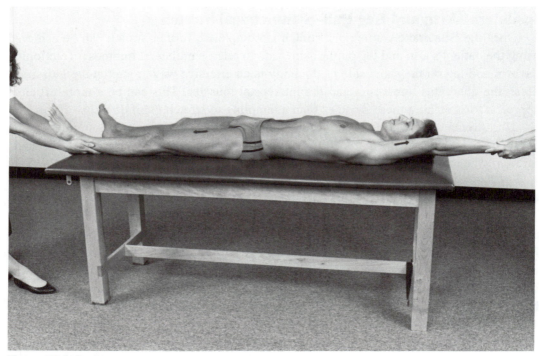

Figure 100A. Supine.

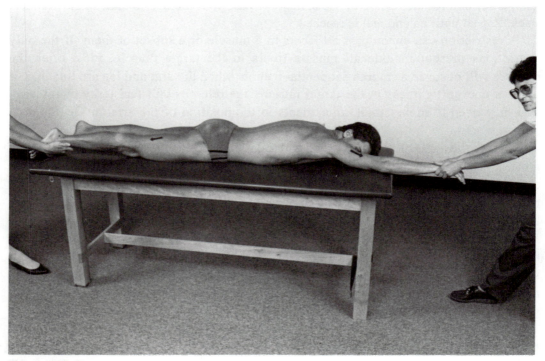

Figure 100B. Prone.

Figure 100. Two person Ipsilateral Arm and Leg Pull.

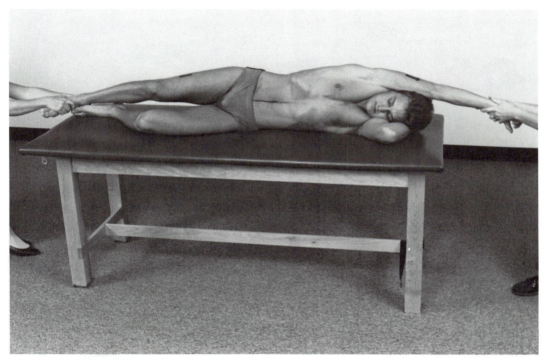

Figure 100C. Side-lying.

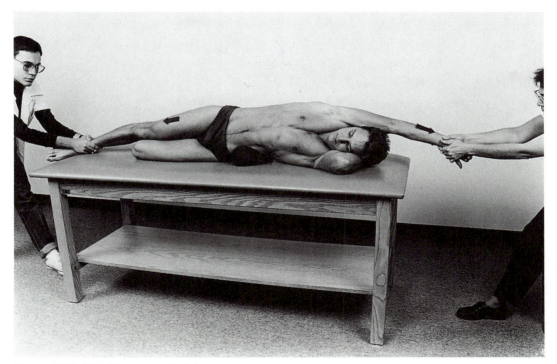

Figure 100D. Side-lying over a bolster.

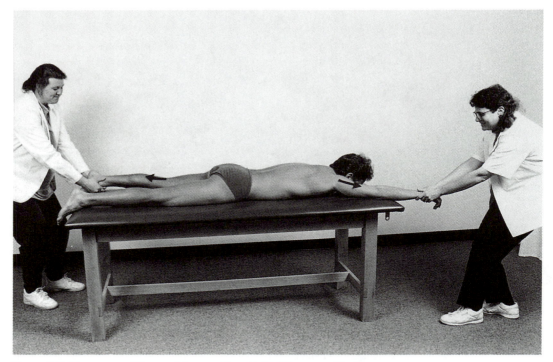

Figure 101. Two person Diagonal Arm and Leg Pull with your patient prone.

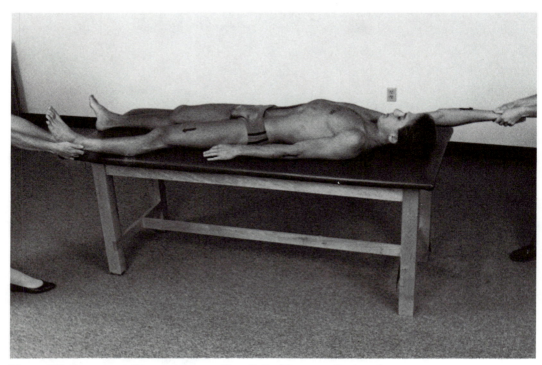

Figure 102. Two person Diagonal Arm and Leg Pull with your patient supine.

Stretching the Pectorals

The pectorals can be placed into an end-range stretch more efficiently using a two person technique after preliminary stretching has released the more superficial restrictions. Have your assistant begin an Arm Pull with your patient's arm aligned with the fibers of the pectorals which you have targeted with your hands (Figures 103 and 104). Maintain your initial stretch of the pectorals, while your assistant releases the remaining excess tension from your patient's arm and shoulder muscles. When your assistant has reached an end feel, increase your stretch to take up the available slack, hold, wait for the release and then stretch again. You will need to direct your assistant to alter the angle of the arm to the body as different fibers of the pectoral muscles are placed in a position of greatest ease to allow the stretch. Continue until an end feel is reached.

As the pectoralis major relaxes, your attention will be drawn to the pectoralis minor. Feedback received through your hands will dictate the position and the amount of traction needed for most efficient stretching.

Stretching the Shoulder Portion of the Upper Trapezius

The shoulder portion of the upper trapezius can be easily stretched in the same way as the pectorals in a two person technique. Have your assistant begin an Arm Pull with your patient's arm aligned with the fibers of the upper trapezius, which you have targeted with your hands (Figure 105). Maintain your initial stretch of the shoulder portion of the upper trapezius while your assistant releases the remaining excess tension from your patient's arm and shoulder joint muscles. When your assistant has reached an end feel, increase your stretch to take up the available slack, hold, wait for the release and then stretch again. You will need to direct your assistant to alter the angle of the arm to the body as different fibers are placed in a position of greatest ease to allow the stretch. Continue until an end feel is reached.

Stretching the Lower Trapezius

With your patient in the prone position, the lower trapezius can be quickly placed into its end range of stretch when your assistant performs either a single or Bilateral Arm Pull. The Bilateral Arm Pull promotes a more symmetrical posture.

Target the lower trapezius with a moderate stretch while your assistant performs an Arm Pull (Figure 106). When your assistant has reached an end feel, increase your stretch to take up the available slack. Hold, wait for the release and then stretch again. Repeat until an end feel is reached and then stretch the other lower trapezius. Finish with a symmetrical stretch by anchoring the distal attachment of both trapezii with one hand. Anchor the proximal attachments by using your hand and forearm (Figure 107).

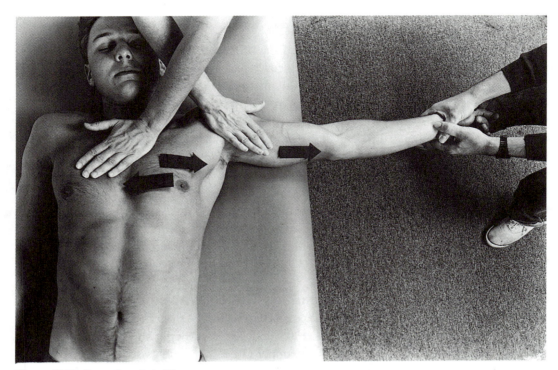

Figure 103A. Cross-hand position.

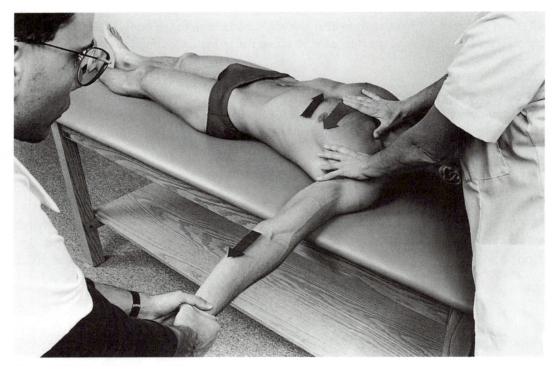

Figure 103B. Straight-hand position.

Figure 103. Two person stretching of the horizontal fibers of the pectoralis major.

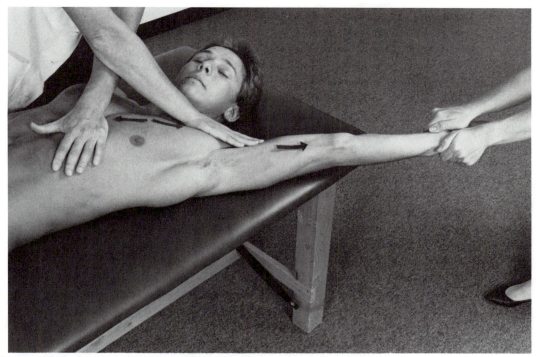

Figure 104. Two person stretching of the lower fibers of the pectoralis major.

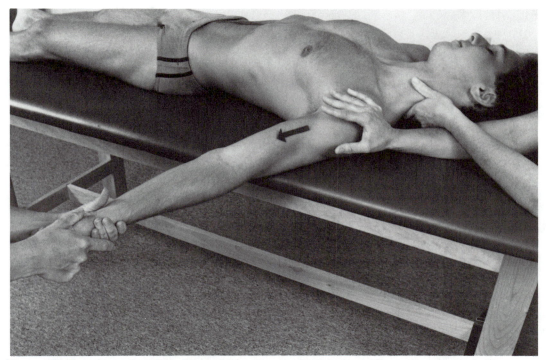

Figure 105. Two person technique for stretching the shoulder portion of the upper trapezius.

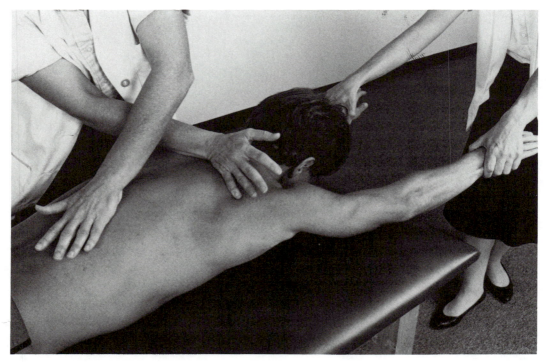

Figure 106. Two person stretching of the lower trapezius.

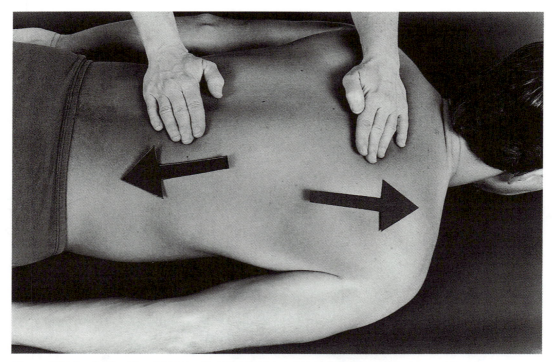

Figure 107. Anchoring the attachments of the the lower trapezii using your hands and forearm.

Three Person Techniques

Additional fine tuning of stretch is possible with three person stretching techniques. While two assistants apply traction to the arms, the legs, or both the arms and legs of the patient, the therapist performs focused stretching to the target muscle(s) in between (see Figures 108-119). Slight alterations in the position of the extremities are used to place the target muscle in the position of greatest ease to allow maximum relaxation. This stretch can be finely focused down to the myofibril level, allowing relaxation unachievable with any other method.

Place your hands on the target muscle and take up the available slack while your assistants apply traction to the arm(s) and leg(s). As they apply traction, you will be able to determine if the arm(s) and leg(s) are at the proper angle to the body to allow the greatest ease of movement. All changes in angle should be performed slowly and smoothly so you can detect any hesitations or skips. As subtle tension is revealed and released, you may need to change your angle of stretch. If spontaneous motion of the arm(s) or leg(s) or both begins, continue stretching the target muscle while your assistants apply enough drag to keep the movement slow and controlled.

Stretching the Shoulder Portion of the Upper Trapezius

Stand or sit behind your patient's head. Place your hands on the shoulder portion of upper trapezii proximal to his shoulder joints, stretching laterally and slightly downward. The line of pull on the arms is determined initially by the slope of your patient's shoulders. As your assistants apply traction on both arms, you will be able to determine the proper line of pull through the proprioceptive feedback you receive from your patient's body (Figure 109). When all the available slack has been taken up, hold and wait for the the excess tension to release. Then stretch again. Repeat until an end feel is reached.

If you detect asymmetrical tightness, you can switch both hands to that portion of the muscle while your assistants continue to apply traction. As the end range is reached, the neck portion of the upper trapezii will be stretched also. By moving your fingers forward in the front of the shoulder joint and increasing your downward pressure, you can begin stretching the diagonal fibers of the pectoralis major.

Stretching the Middle Trapezius

The middle trapezii are not often targeted for stretching because they are overstretched by anterior chest wall tightness. However, stretching the middle trapezii is sometimes necessary to allow stretching of muscles which lie beneath it.

Place your crossed hands on the distal attachments of the middle trapezii and stretch to take up the slack while your assistants apply traction equally to both arms along the direction of the muscle fibers (Figure 110). Hold until the release occurs and stretch again. Direct your assistants to either increase the traction, to maintain steady traction or release the traction depending upon the feedback you are receiving. Sometimes you will want to increase your stretch and other times you will want your assistants to increase theirs. Repeat until an end feel is reached.

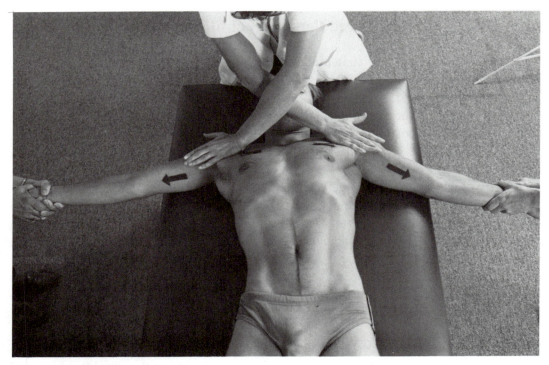

Figure 108A. Cross-hand technique.

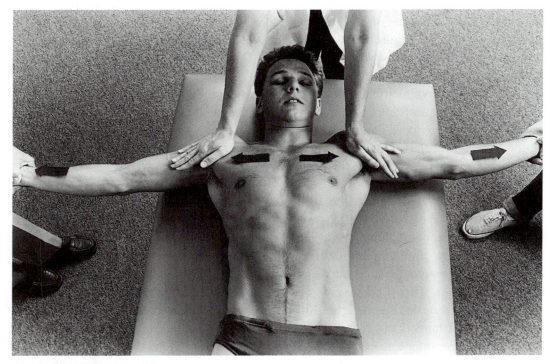

Figure 108B. Straight-hand technique.

Figure 108. Three person technique for stretching the horizontal fibers of the pectoralis major.

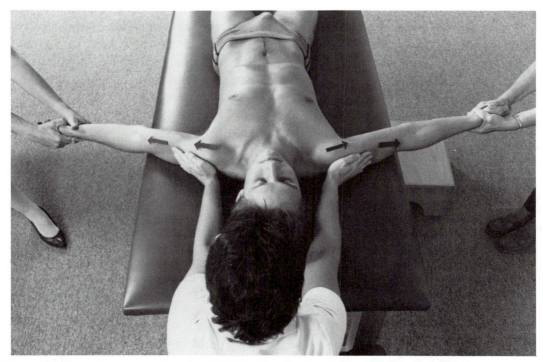

Figure 109. Three person technique for stretching the shoulder portion of the upper trapezii.

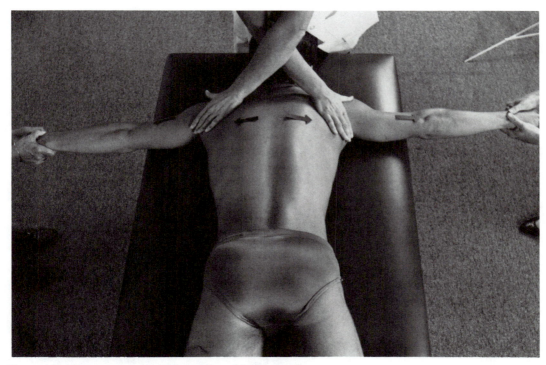

Figure 110. Three person stretching of the middle trapezii.

When focusing attention on the middle trapezii, the arms should be perpendicular to the body with little tendency to move. However, as soon as the restrictions in the middle trapezius muscle are released, you may find your hands drawn to stretch deeper restrictions. Direct your assistants to maintain a steady traction. The line of pull will then correspond to the uncovered restrictions.

Arm and Leg Pull with Focused Stretching

Tractioning the arm and leg on the same side of the body is a very effective means of anchoring muscles which are difficult to approach directly, such as the latissimus dorsi and the erector spinae with their multiple attachments, the intercostals, and the quadratus laborum with its proximal attachment on the the lower ribs. The therapist can perform focused stretching on the most restricted area within a long muscle, such as the erector spinae, while the Arm and Leg Pull anchor the entire muscle group (Figure 111).

This stretch can be performed with the patient prone, supine or side-lying depending upon the target muscle. Multiple variations of side-lying can be used to further isolate the target muscle.

Latissimus Dorsi

The latissimus dorsi presents a unique stretching problem with its multiple attachments at the pelvis, the ribs, the scapula and the upper arm. Using the Arm and Leg Pull to anchor this muscle will allow the therapist to identify and stretch its more restricted areas before stretching the muscle as a whole.

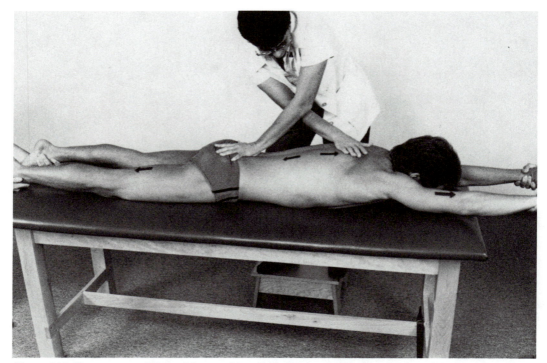

Figure 111. Three person Bilateral Arm and Leg Pull with longitudinal stretching of the erector spinae.

Begin stretching with your patient supine on the plinth. Using crossed hands, start stretching with your hands far apart while your assistants apply traction to your patient's ipsilateral arm and leg (Figure 112). Hold until a release is felt and stretch again. As areas of increased restriction are located, focus your stretching on those areas while directing the line and force of pull from your assistants (Figure 113). Repeat until an end feel is reached in this position.

Without changing your position, have your assistants switch to a concave stretch using Bilateral Arm and Leg Pulls (Figure 114). If additional areas of increased restriction are located, perform focused stretching. If no additional restrictions are located, stretch the latissimus dorsi as a whole.

The side-lying ipsilateral stretch further stretches the latissimus dorsi into a position of maximum stretch. Change from the concave stretch back to a straight stretch and roll your patient onto his side. Once he is on his side, instruct your assistants to resume the ipsilateral stretch, angling the arm and leg down toward the floor (Figure 115). For additional stretch or to eliminate the indentation of the waist, a bolster can be placed under your patient's side. Continue stretching by first stretching the muscle as a whole and then stretching focused areas of restriction. End with stretching the entire muscle again until an end feel is reached in all areas. It is imperative to stretch both latissimus dorsi in the same treatment session in order to prevent your patient from feeling disoriented and asymmetrical.

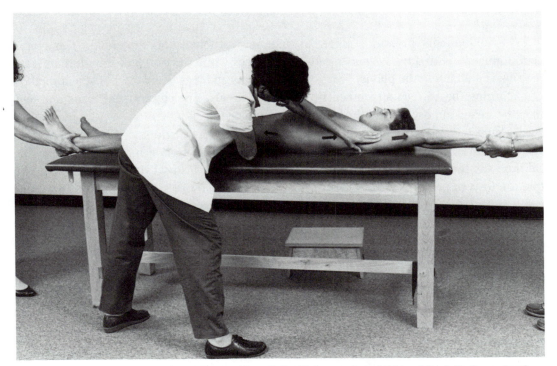

Figure 112. Three person Ipsilateral Arm and Leg Pull with focused stretching of the latissimus dorsi.

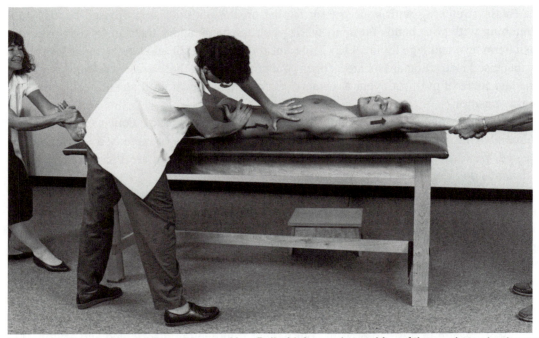

Figure 113. Three person Ipsilateral Arm and Leg Pull with focused stretching of the quadratus lumborum and the overlying latissimus dorsi.

Abdominals

The abdominals present a different anatomic problem for stretching. The rectus abdominus is divided by a ligamentous aponeuroses while the obliques interdigitate with the ribs and attach to the pelvis. Traction on the arms and legs is the only efficient method of anchoring the various attachments of the abdominals. The angle of the arms and legs must be varied almost constantly as stretching proceeds.

Be sure to ask your patient to empty his bladder before beginning this stretch. Begin stretching the rectus abdominus with crossed hands, placing one hand proximal to the sternum and the other at the symphysis pubis (Figure 116). Instruct your assistants to apply traction to your patient's arms and legs to take up the available slack. Hold until a release is felt and stretch again. As areas of increased restriction are located, focus your stretching on those areas while directing your assistants' line and force of pull. Repeat until an end feel is reached and your hands are back in your starting position.

Change your hand position to the obliques while instructing your assistants to perform the complementary contralateral stretch (Figure 117). Alter your assistants' positions until the obliques are in the position of greatest ease. Hold until a release is felt and stretch again. Repeat until an end feel is reached. Then alter the angle of the arm and leg a few degrees to determine if further tightness is present. As areas of increased restriction are located, perform focused stretching while directing your assistants' line and force of traction. Repeat until an end feel is reached and the entire myofascial unit is stretched. Repeat on the opposite diagonal.

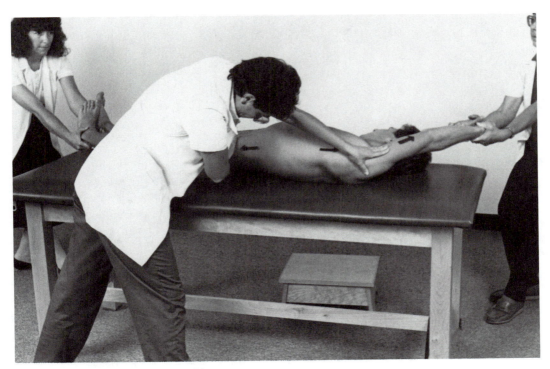

Figure 114A. View from the convex side.

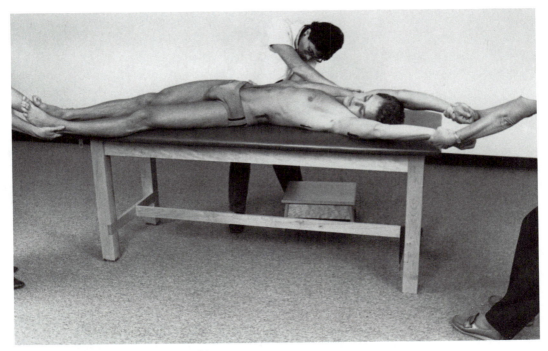

Figure 114B. View from the concave side.

Figure 114. Three person concave Bilateral Arm and Leg Pull with focused stretching of the latissimus dorsi.

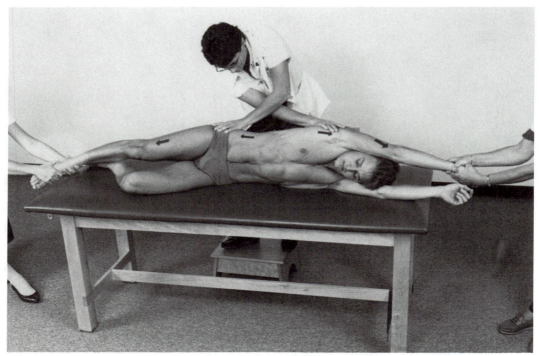

Figure 115. Three person side-lying Arm and Leg Pull with focused stretching of the latissimus dorsi.

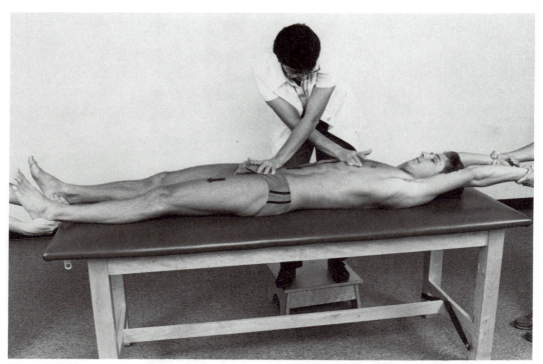

Figure 116. Three person straight Bilateral Arm and Leg Pulls with focused stretching of the abdominal muscles.

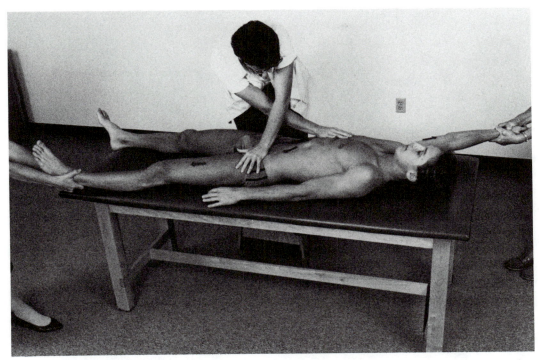

Figure 117. Three person Contralateral Arm and Leg Pull with focused stretching of the oblique muscles.

Once all the tightness of the obliques is released, stretch the rectus abdominus again while your assistants perform Bilateral Arm and Leg Pulls. If any localized tightness remains, perform focused stretching and then return to your starting hand position for a final stretch.

Erector Spinae

Although it is made up of several different muscles which interdigitate with each other and with the spinous processes, the erector spinae is usually treated as one myofascial unit. Begin stretching with your hands crossed and widely separated while your assistants perform Bilateral Arm and Leg Pulls (see Figure 111). Hold until a release occurs and stretch again. Continue until an end feel is reached. As areas of restriction are located, perform focused stretching while directing your assistants' angle of stretch. As each local restriction is placed in its position of greatest ease, the restriction should release in a smooth flowing motion. Change your position by only a few degrees as you seek other restrictions. When no further focused stretching is possible, repeat your long stretch.

Without changing your position, have your assistants switch to a concave stretch using Bilateral Arm and Leg Pulls (Figure 118). Perform focused stretching on any additional areas of increased restriction. Repeat in the opposite direction. When no additional restrictions are located, stretch the erector spinae as a whole.

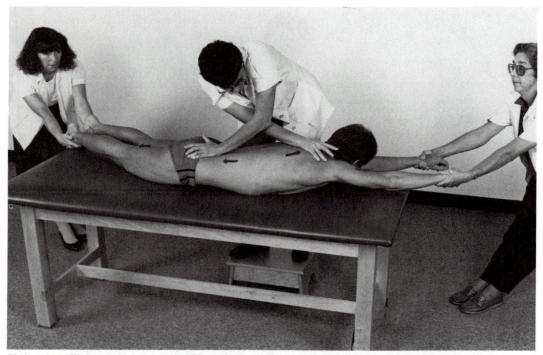

Figure 118. Three person concave Bilateral Arm and Leg Pulls with focused stretching of the erector spinae.

Change your position to an oblique stretch while instructing your assistants to perform the complementary contralateral stretch (Figure 119). Although this corresponds with no known anatomic structure other than fascia, it is an effective stretch clinically. As areas of localized restrictions become obvious, perform focused stretching while directing your assistants' angle of stretch. Continue until an end feel is reached. When no additional restrictions are located, perform a final stretch with your hands in your original oblique position. Repeat on the opposite diagonal. When no further restrictions are located, finish by stretching the entire erector spinae in a straight position one last time.

Trigger Points

Active myofascial trigger points are discrete, reproducible foci of hypersensitivity. When palpated, trigger points result in localized sharp pain, radiating pain and referred pain.[19,30-43] This pain rarely, if ever, follows dermatomal or peripheral nerve distribution patterns.[19,44] Myofascial trigger point pain patterns are well documented.[19,30,35,45-65]

Active myofascial trigger points are painful without stimulation. An active myofascial trigger point is always sensitive, restricts motion,[19,40,66-71] causes muscle weakness,[40,63] elicits protective muscle spasm with an adequate stimulus and often produces predictable autonomic responses. These autonomic responses can include vasoconstriction, vasodilatation, hypersecretion, global hypersensitivity and pain either locally or distally with adequate stimulation.[19,30,36,40,63,71-75] Myofascial trigger points are areas of lowered skin

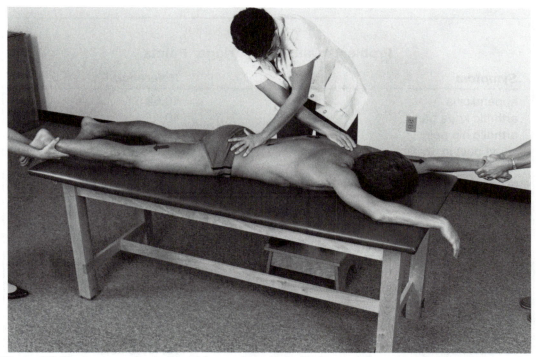

Figure 119. Three person Contralateral Arm and Leg Pull with focused diagonal stretching of the erector spinae.

resistance [74] and sometimes are associated with fibrositic nodules.[31,32,76,77] Trigger points may elicit the "jump sign" with palpation.[35,40,78]

Active myofascial trigger points can cause secondary trigger points in agonistic and antagonistic muscles. These trigger points develop in response to overload, as these muscles try to compensate for or assist the injured muscle by splinting. Satellite trigger points can develop within the reference zone of the original active trigger point.[19] Latent trigger points are painful only with palpation [19,40,67,68] and may elicit the same sensory, autonomic and motor phenomena with an adequate stimulus.

As hyperexcitable foci, myofascial trigger points respond to increasingly smaller stimuli over time.[19,30,40,79] Thus, patients who complain of increasing pain are reporting a real phenomenon and are not simply becoming chronic complainers.

Often myofascial trigger points are found in a taut band of skeletal muscle or fascia.[19,36,39,40,71,77,80] Trigger points can be found in scar tissue,[81] tendons, ligaments, skin, fat pads, joint capsules and periosteum. Trigger points which are not myofascial in origin are local irritants and do not cause related autonomic, sensory, or motor phenomena or the referred pain patterns. These trigger points must be released to allow maximum relaxation of all restricted tissues and eradication of the localized pain.

Myofascial trigger points can cause or mimic many different problems. These problems defy diagnosis since they do not respond positively to the standard diagnostic tests or treatment for that problem. However, elimination of the myofascial trigger point will also completely eliminate the problem. Some of these problems are listed in Table 3-1. The complaints listed in the table are the indications for Myofascial Release when no other

Table 3-1.
Problems Caused By Trigger Points

Symptom	Reference
appendicitis	40,56
arthritic knee pain	40
arthritic hip pain	40
chest pain in atypical anginal patterns	19,34,40,46,53,82,83
diarrhea	84
dizziness	19
dysmenorrhea	40
epicondylitis	19,40,69
facial neuralgia, atypical	19,40,62,85,86
fibromyositis	34
heel spur	40,59,69
hiccups	87
inguinal pain	88
jaw/TMJ pain	52,66-68,85,89
muscle spasm	19
occipital neuralgia	19,40,85,90,91
sciatica	35,40,55,59
subdeltoid bursitis	19,37,40,92
tension headache	19,35,40,46,85,90
thoracic inlet syndrome	19,35,40,46,55,85
tooth pain	19
tinnitus	65
torticollis, acute	19,40,93
trochanteric bursitis	40,59
vertigo	19,94
vomiting, uncontrollable	19

physical reason is found for the complaint. For example, the patient with angina-like pain and no known underlying cardiac cause may have tightness in the chest wall and active myofascial trigger points. Following a Myofascial Arm Pull and Trigger Point Releases, the angina-like pain will be eliminated.

Successfully treated medical problems may leave myofascial tightness that also responds quite effectively to myofascial stretching. Trigger points within mature scar tissue and the scar itself need to be released to eliminate restrictions caused by adhesions and to allow free movement. Although the release sensation is quite painful and perceived as knife-like and tearing, no reopening of the wound occurs. The release of restriction gives back movement the patient was unaware of losing. Problems distal to, and seemingly unrelated to, a scar can be alleviated by treatment of the scar.

There is a reflex relationship between muscles that are under tension due to trigger points. Release of a trigger point in one muscle may, through reflex inhibition, also relax other muscles which are exhibiting increased tension. For example, relaxation of the gluteus maximus may eliminate pain and tenderness referred to the coccyx or the levator ani. Release of the suboccipital muscles may relax the sternocleidomastoid, and vice versa, while release of the thoracolumbar erector spinae muscles may relax the iliopsoas. The sternocleidomastoid and the scalene muscles reciprocally affect the pectoral muscles.[69,95]

Latent and active myofascial trigger points prevent maximal relaxation of the myofascial unit. These myofascial trigger points must be released in conjunction with myofascial stretching before a true end point is achieved. Maximal elongation does not occur when trigger points are present. When the myofascial unit returns to its pre-treatment length within minutes, hours or several days, all of the trigger points within it are not released. Therefore, even if the patient does not complain of point tenderness, less than optimal relaxation and stretching of the myofascial unit suggests that untreated or incompletely treated trigger points are present.

When no further trigger points are found within a specific myofascial unit but the stretch does not hold, other distal trigger points may be maintaining tension in the target myofascial unit. Alternatively, dural tube restrictions may be maintaining the abnormal tension. The differential diagnosis of the locus of the restriction depends upon the speed at which the tension returns. If the pain was totally eliminated during a treatment session and tension returns immediately at the end of the session, dural tube restrictions are present.

Trigger Point Releases

Many different treatments have been used to eliminate trigger points with varying results. These include reflex inhibition following minimal or maximal isometric contraction,[69,85] ultrasound,[96] neuroprobe, electro-acuscope, dry needling,[48,63,97,98] anesthetic blocks,[30,47,54,55,64,65,88] intense cold,[30,56,62,63,85,94,99] TENS,[54] infrared,[97] massage,[100] and ischemic pressure.[101] No one technique has emerged which is superior to the others. Perpetuating factors such as vitamin deficiencies and underlying organic disease make the ultimate elimination of trigger points even more difficult.[19] Myofascial stretching should be part of a multifaceted approach to trigger point treatment.

Melzack found that 71% of acupuncture points used to treat pain corresponded with myofascial trigger points.[54] An acupuncture chart can help the therapist begin to locate trigger points. A knowledge of trigger points and their radiation patterns will help the therapist understand complicated pain complaints. Both volumes of *Myofascial Pain and Dysfunction: The Trigger Point Manual* by Janet Travell and David Simons[19,102] describe the primary trigger points and their radiation patterns and are valuable texts for both therapist and patient.

I ask my patients to look at the illustrations in both volumes and place markers on the ones which duplicate their pain complaint. I encourage my patients to read as much as they want in these books. Frequently, my patients will thank me for showing them their pain complaints are real and not "all in their head."

Much of my treatment is focused on elimination of trigger points or the relegation of trigger points to latent status. Release of the primary trigger point not only eliminates that trigger point but also eliminates the secondary and satellite ones, along with the associated sensory, motor and autonomic phenomena.[19] The trigger points that are released visit after visit and return almost before the patient leaves the treatment room are secondary or satellite points. Only when the primary trigger points are identified and released and the perpetuating factors eliminated will lasting relief be gained by the patient.

Muscle relaxants temporarily eliminate secondary and satellite trigger points. Because splinting is eliminated by muscle relaxants, there is a temporary exacerbation of pain from the primary trigger points.[19] A single dose of a muscle relaxant approximately two hours before assessment will allow mapping of primary trigger points. Whenever possible, treatment is directed at the primary trigger points. However, a trigger point can be primary for one pain pattern and be reinforced as a secondary or satellite trigger point in another overlapping pattern. Thus, a simplistic or reductionistic approach to trigger points is not appropriate.

Treat the most recent injury and its trigger points first and then proceed backward to older injuries and related trigger points. The number of treatments required is determined by the severity and age of the injuries. In general, the older the injury, the more secondary and satellite trigger points there are, the more global the pain pattern will be, and the longer the treatment will take.

The initial goal of treatment is to localize the pain pattern and more sharply define the location of the trigger points causing or existing within the pain pattern. As this puzzle is unraveled, your patient will be able to assist more actively in the localization and elimination of the trigger points that are the primary pain generators. You will be directed to these trigger points by feedback from your patient's body. The altered tissue tension acts like a magnet which will hold your attention until the trigger point has been neutralized and is no longer a pain focus.

Trigger points can be layered and must be released sequentially in a relatively straight downward movement. They can also be proximal to each other. As each trigger point is released, your fingers will be drawn laterally and downward from layer to layer until the final trigger point is eliminated.

Trigger points are released manually by carefully graded increasing pressure using one finger (Figure 120), several fingers (Figure 121), the knuckles (Figure 122), or an elbow (Figure 123). The variations are limited only by the therapist's ingenuity and coordination. On occasion more than one point will need to be released at the same time to break up a feedback pattern.

When a trigger point is palpated, the surrounding tissue tension will increase. Increasing pressure on the trigger point causes radiation of the pain pattern. As the pain sensation intensifies, the patient's original pain complaint may be duplicated.

Trigger Point Releases follow the same pattern as other Myofascial Releases. The initial pressure takes up the available slack in the surrounding tissue albeit in a downward or inward direction. As the trigger point gradually relaxes, the pressure is increased to take up the additional slack. Your fingers will be drawn to other trigger points by the alteration in tissue tension in the deeper body layers. Most often you will find your finger being drawn inward in a spiral pattern.

Feedback from the patient directs your treatment. You work in concert and rhythm with the patient's body, increasing pressure as needed and easing back as needed. As the layers of the trigger point release, your hand is pulled more deeply into the restricted tissues. At the point of final and total release of the trigger point, your patient may also experience an

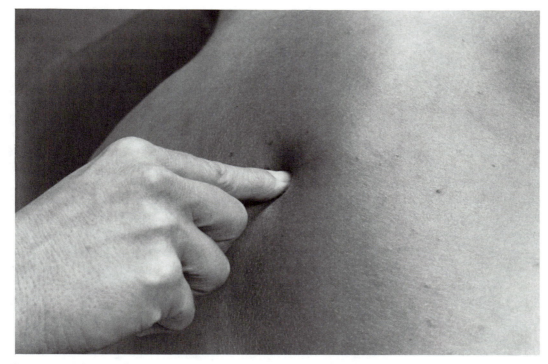

Figure 120. Using one finger for ischemic pressure on a myofascial trigger point.

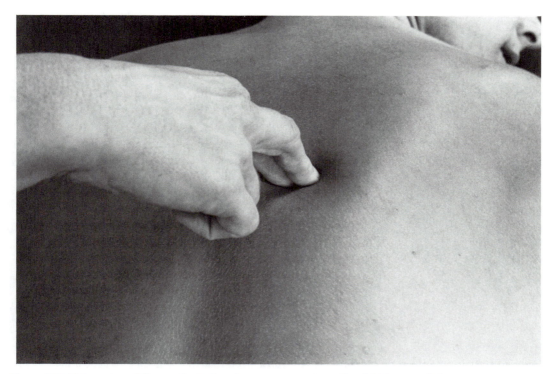

Figure 121. Using several fingers for ischemic pressure on a myofascial trigger point.

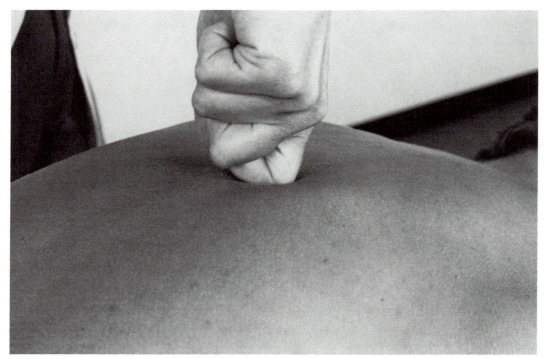

Figure 122. Using a knuckle for ischemic pressure on a myofascial trigger point.

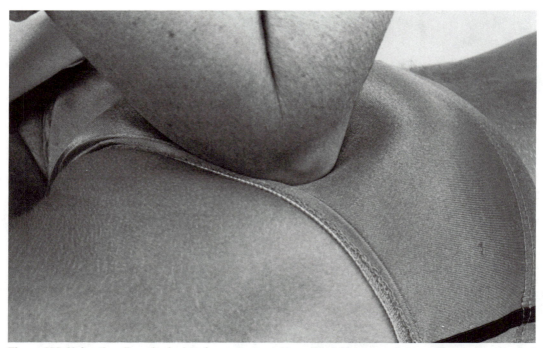

Figure 123. Using the elbow for ischemic pressure on a myofascial trigger point on a deeper muscle such as the piriformis.

emotional release.[15,16,103] As the altered tissue tension slowly disappears, you will feel your hand being released from the trigger point's grip. However, another nearby trigger point may claim your immediate attention and start the cycle anew with little pause.

Prior to a Trigger Point Release, I tell my patient that the release will be painful but limited. I encourage my patient to express the pain verbally or to let the tears flow. Each person has his own style of releasing tension and pain. I do not take personally anything said during a Trigger Point Release. This expression can be very abusive and negative as my patient's pain increases and peaks. Shutting off this emotional expression is counterproductive.

Your patients will recognize the need and efficacy of this treatment if all previous attempts at eliminating the trigger point(s) have had limited or no success. I always tell my patients I will stop if they want me to but none has ever done so. The sensation is one of a "good hurt," necessary but painful. The whole key to successful Trigger Point Releasing lies in being able to allow feedback from the patient to direct treatment and to convey your empathy and caring through touch.

Release of trigger points must be considered a deep and painful technique. Although Trigger Point Releases are patient-guided, intially most patients will have little active participation in the release. When using deep pressure to release the trigger points, the patient must be given an "out word" and permission to stop the release if the pain becomes intolerable. First explain to the patient that if he can allow the pain to increase and reach maximum intensity, the release will be more complete and will allow the greatest amount of relaxation of the myofascial tissues. Two or more sessions may be needed to completely eradicate the long-standing trigger points.

Once your patient understands the process of Trigger Point Releases, he will be able to become a more active participant in the process. As you locate a trigger point, your patient will be able to recognize the radiation pattern from it. A patient who has good body awareness and control will be able to relax the tissue surrounding the trigger point when you begin to apply pressure to it. Some patients will be able to drop the surrounding tissue tension so low that a complete Trigger Point Release occurs. Since it begins in the deepest tissues and moves outward, this is the most efficient Trigger Point Release.

Scar Releases

Scars limit movement through superficial and deep adhesions. Just like active myofascial trigger points, scars limit releases. No matter which direction you approach from, you are always stopped at the scar. If the scar cannot be released, you have hit the anatomic limit of what you can do to facilitate your patient's most efficient movement pattern.

Assess scar movement in the same way as superficial skin restrictions. If the scar is in a broad skin area, assess movement with the palm of your hand (Figure 124) or by Skin Rolling (see Figure 88). In smaller areas, use one finger to move the scar or use a modified Skin Roll by pinching the scar between your thumb and second finger.

Due to the intense pain it causes the patient, release of scars must be considered a deep release technique no matter which method is used. Your patient will tell you that a scar

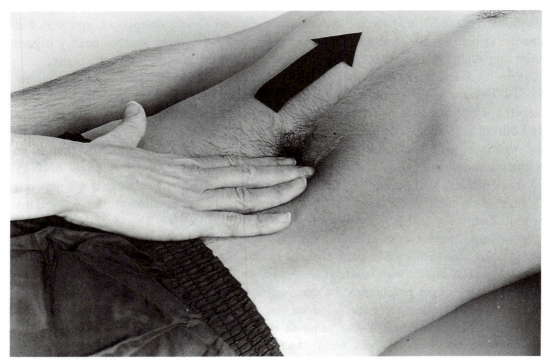

Figure 124A. Upward.

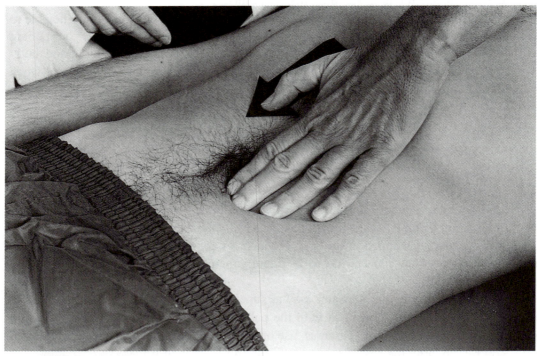

Figure 124B. Downward.

Figure 124. Testing for scar mobility using the entire hand.

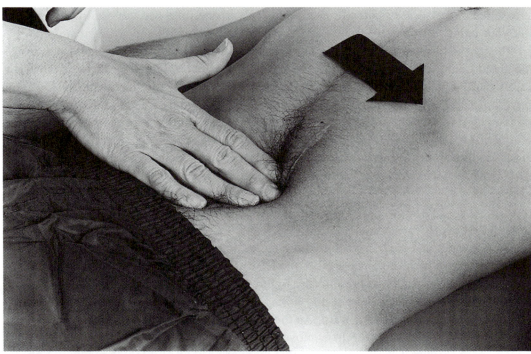

Figure 124C. Left. Note restriction as the skin is bunched in front of the therapist's fingers.

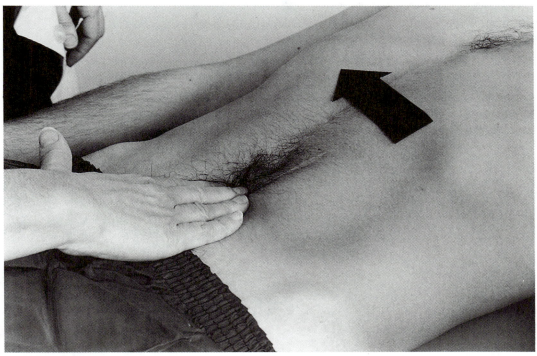

Figure 124D. Right.

release feels like surgery without anesthesia. This is one time you will definitely need to talk your patient through the pain, making it clear that you will stop when requested.

The age of the scar does not affect its potential for being released. Any healed scar can and should be released since it limits the movement of other tissues throughout the body. Rarely will you be able to achieve a full scar release during one treatment session. You may be limited by your patient's pain tolerance or by the body's need to adjust slowly to the increased movement in the area. You may need to repeat these releases during another treatment session(s) until the maximum available release is achieved. Even though an end feel is reached during a treatment session, the Scar Release should be repeated at least one more time to determine if any deeper adhesions are present and are now accessible to release.

Scar Skin Roll

For a given scar, use the least forceful release first. Start with Skin Rolling. If you have enough area in which to work, use both hands rolling the skin up, down and diagonally until no further restriction is present (see Figure 88).

If the scar is deeply adherent and does not move enough to roll, use a pincer grip (Figure 125) to lift the scar upward. As the scar releases, distract the skin upward until no further slack is available. Then, move the skin to the left, wait for the release and stretch again (Figure 126). Continue in this manner until an end feel is reached. Repeat, moving the skin to the right. You may also need to stretch on a diagonal. When no

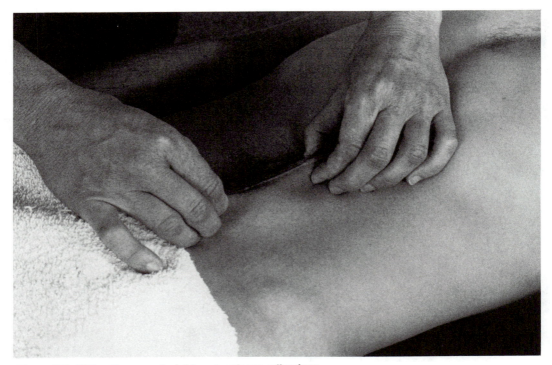

Figure 125. Lifting the scar straight up to release adhesions.

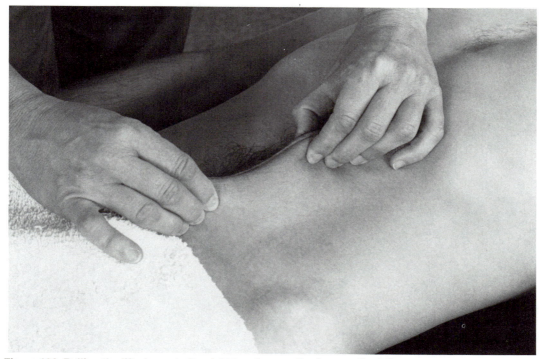

Figure 126. Pulling the lifted scar to the right to release adhesions on the left.

further release is available, again attempt to roll the scar in a Skin Roll to determine if all of the adhesion is released or if deeper adhesions are now accessible to release.

The Scar Skin Roll is a good final technique to use to verify that all restrictions have been eliminated no matter which scar release technique is used.

Indirect Scar Release

Even a deeply indented scar, such as one from a healed abscess, can be released in the same manner in which a muscle is stretched. Place your hands on either side of the scar (Figure 127). Stretch the skin between your hands by moving your hands away from each other until no further movement is possible. Hold until a release is felt and then stretch again. When no further stretch is possible in that direction, reposition your hands so you are stretching the scar at a right angle to your original line of stretch (Figure 128). Proceed as before. If the scar is not completely released, move your hands 45 degrees away from your previous line of stretch and repeat the release procedure until an end feel is reached or the scar is fully mobile (Figure 129).

Direct Scar Release

Stroke slowly along the length of the scar while asking your patient to identify the most sensitive point in that scar (Figure 130). Use enough pressure to keep contact with that point (Figure 131) while rotating your palpating finger in a clockwise direction, again asking your patient to identify the most sensitive point (Figure 132).

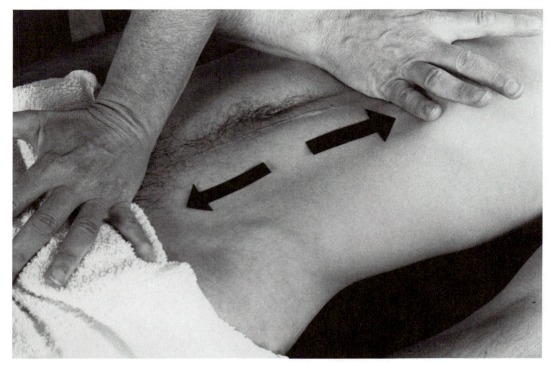

Figure 127. Longitudinal stretching of a scar.

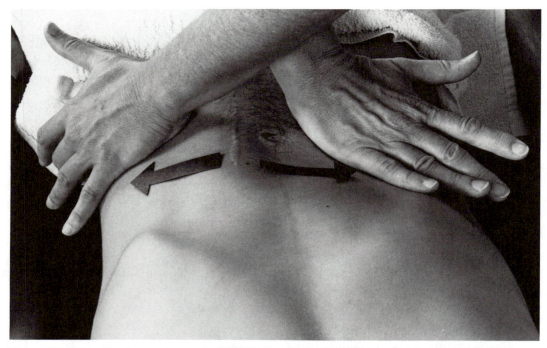

Figure 128. After achieving maximum stretch in the longitudinal direction, repeat the stretch at a 90 degree angle from the original stretch.

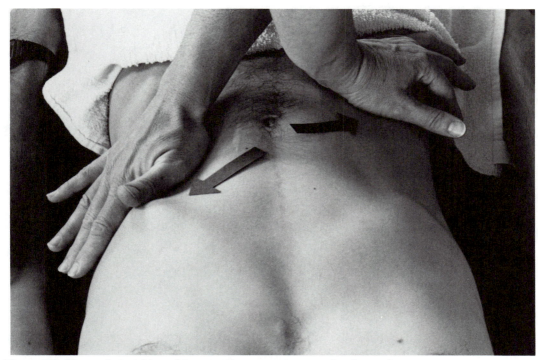

Figure 129. Diagonal stretching of the scar. Repeat on the opposite diagonal.

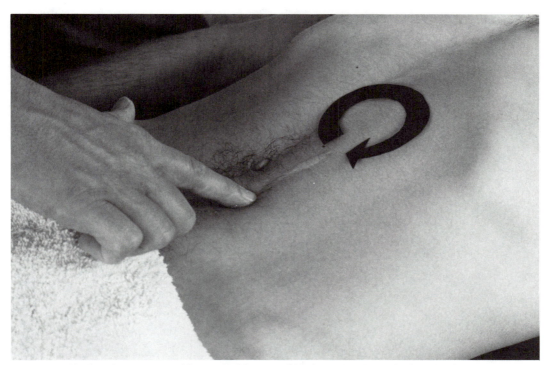

Figure 130. Finding the most sensitive part of the scar. Slowly stroke the entire length of the scar several times, asking your patient to tell you each time where the scar is the most sensitive.

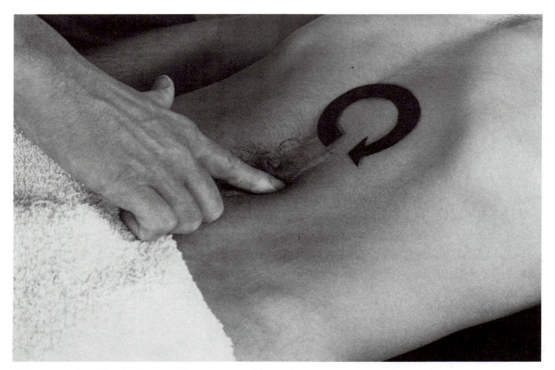

Figure 131. Once having located the most sensitive point, apply just enough pressure to keep your finger from slipping off that point.

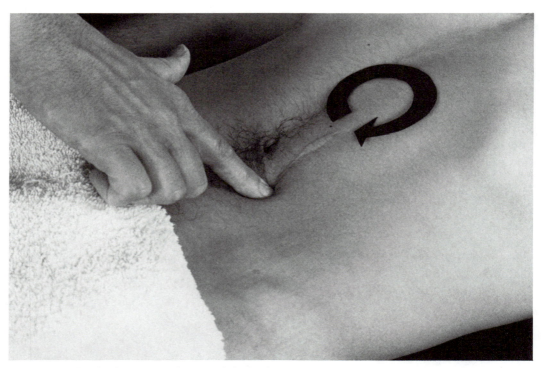

Figure 132. Keeping in contact with the original point, draw the scar around in a circle, again asking your patient to locate the most sensitive point.

Now proceed as with a Trigger Point Release (Figure 133) by using adequate pressure to take up the available slack and allowing your finger to be led into the deeper tissues.[81] Your patient will complain of increasing, severe, and/or cutting pain until the release occurs. At this point he may ask if you have released your pressure when, in fact, you have not. Reactive hyperemia may occur along with a release of heat. Infrequently, the area may become very cold. Slowly release your pressure when no further releases occur.

The end feel is slightly different after this deep release. You will feel a deep calm coming from your patient. He may feel tired and want to sleep for a while before getting up. If this occurs, cover your patient so he stays warm and let him rest quietly.

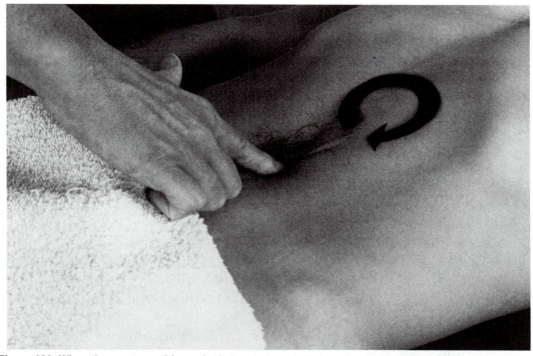

Figure 133. When the most sensitive point is located, apply increasing pressure following the inherent tissue motion until your patient reports a decrease in pain although you have not decreased your pressure.

Strumming

Strumming is a very forceful and painful deep release technique. I consider this to be a technique of last resort to be used only after all myofascial tightness has been released and ligamentous restrictions are preventing further improvement in alignment. Like J Stroking, this technique is not guided by feedback. Unlike J Stroking, there is a real danger of overstretching and causing a ligamentous tear.

Before beginning, explain to your patient why you want to use this technique and the level of pain he will experience. Give your patient an "out word" to use if the pain is more than he is willing or able to tolerate. Generally speaking, athletes are the only people who are willing to experience this pain level to gain an additional few degrees of movement.

Strumming can be used to improve patellar tracking, finish releasing the iliopsoas, break up long-standing hypomobility of one or more vertebrae, and to increase abduction at the hip joint. Strumming can be used around any joint at the end of the available range to achieve full anatomic range of motion when no other reason for decrease range other than ligamentous tightness is present.

Strumming is similar to a connective tissue massage technique[28] and to Rolfing.[9] When used as a Myofascial Release technique, Strumming is used in a very limited body area after all soft tissue releases have been achieved.

Strumming is very tiring for your hands. Do not attempt to perform it longer than thirty to sixty seconds until you build up a tolerance for this technique. Your patient may not tolerate even thirty seconds of Strumming initially.

I prefer to treat my patients with interferential TENS and ice to prevent swelling and to decrease pain after using Strumming. If my patient does not tolerate ice, I use moist heat and interferential TENS.

Short Duration, Strong Strumming

Strumming is usually performed with the fingers held in rigid extension with or without flexion at the metacarpal phalangeal joints (Figures 134 and 135). Position yourself for optimum leverage. Apply pressure gradually to the restricted site either perpendicular to or parallel to the ligamentous fibers. Once all of the slack is taken up, use a back and forth scrubbing motion while maintaining your pressure. As releases occur, you will need to gradually increase your pressure to keep the tissues taut. Continue until a end feel is reached or your patient tells you to stop.

Alternately, you may cup your hand into a claw-like position (Figure 136) and use a windshield wiper motion with deep pressure across or perpendicular to the ligamentous insertion of the myofascial unit. This technique is particularly useful along the rim of the pelvis.

Long Stroke Strumming

A milder and more tolerable form of Strumming is long slow stroking, which is used over long muscle bellies. This form of Strumming is performed using the elbows (Figure 137) or knuckles (Figure 138). As you stroke slowly down the muscle belly, sequential releases occur. Keep the onion metaphor in mind as you stroke deeper with each subsequent pass down the muscle. This type of Strumming is useful in the

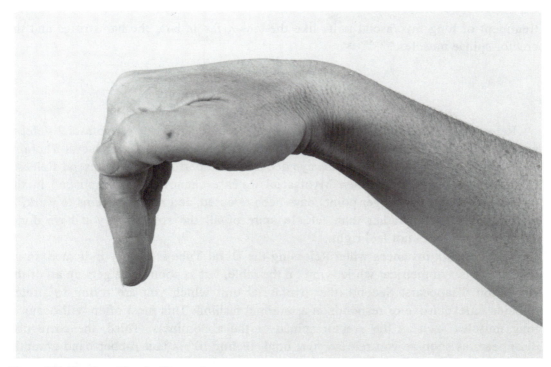

Figure 134. Hand position for Strumming.

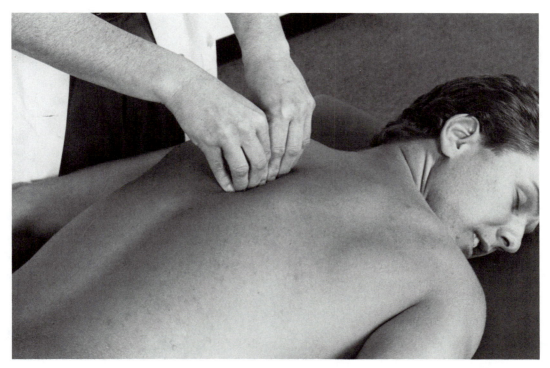

Figure 135. Strumming the thoracic erector spinae as it inserts into the lateral border of the spinal column.

treatment of long myofascial units like the tensor fascia lata, the hamstrings and the erector spinae muscles.

Releasing the Dural Tube

Releasing the Dural Tube is the connecting technique between Myofascial Release and Craniosacral Therapy. While it is an essential element in Craniosacral Therapy, Releasing the Dural Tube is not always needed when performing Myofascial Release. However, there are times when Myofascial Release cannot be accomplished in the usual manner. All the trigger points have been released, and nothing seems to work. A restriction is sensed rather than felt. In spite of all the stretching you have done, something just does not feel right.

There are six instances when Releasing the Dural Tube is clearly indicated. First, the patient is symmetrical while lying on the table, but as soon as he gets up all of the correction disappears. Second, the myofascial unit which you are trying to stretch remains unresponsive or responds in a minimal fashion. This most often will occur in long muscles such as the erector spinae or the abdominals. Third, the correction disappears as soon as you release your hold, feeling like a taut rubber band abruptly returning to its non-stretched length. This is most likely to occur following an Occipital Base Release. Fourth, you perceive a feeling through your hands that something still needs to be released, but you are unable to identify the specific structure. Fifth, as mentioned earlier, the patient is pain-free following treatment, but the pain returns

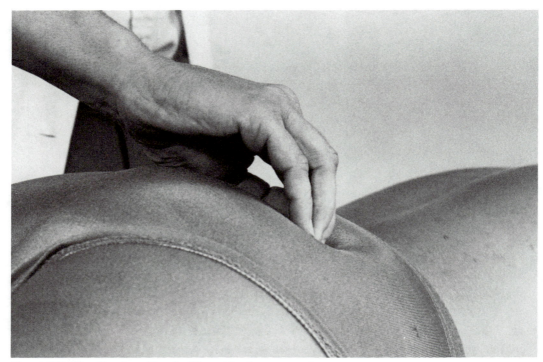

Figure 136. Claw hand position for Strumming larger muscle groups.

almost immediately. Sixth, Trigger Point Releases are successful in eliminating secondary, satellite and tertiary trigger points, but it does not last. Releasing the Dural Tube in these situations makes the difference between a successful treatment session and an unsuccessful one.

For example, I was working with a patient who had active myofascial trigger points and myofascial restrictions in the abdomen in addition to chronic neck and low back pain. Manual Trigger Point Releases were only partially successful, as was using spray and stretch techniques. My assistant and I tried a two person longitudinal stretch and were unable to relax the abdominal muscles. They remained taut and unyielding until we released the dural tube. When the dural tube was released, the abdominal muscles relaxed in a wave-like manner immediately after we resumed the longitudinal stretch.

There is no explanation for how or why Releasing the Dural Tube works. This technique is completely indirect, and its effectiveness is measured by your patient's report of increased comfort or reduced pain. Clinically, once you have perfected the technique there will be no question that the technique works.

Anatomy of the Dural Membrane System

The brain is soft and gelatinous, while the spinal cord is of a slightly firmer consistency. The meninges, skull and vertebral column with its associated ligaments protect the central nervous system. These associated ligaments consist of the dura mater which is the thick outer layer lined by the more delicate arachnoid and the thin pia mater. The pia mater adheres to the surfaces of the brain and spinal cord. In addition, the pia mater and the arachnoid line the subarachnoid space which is filled with the cerebrospinal fluid.

The dura mater and the cerebrospinal fluid provide the main support and protection of the brain and the spinal cord. The cranial dura mater is attached to the periosteum lining the internal surfaces of the skull. This periosteum is continuous with the periosteum on the external surface of the skull, at the margins of the foramen magnum and the smaller foramina for the nerves and blood vessels.[104]

The cranial dura mater is a dense firm layer of collagenous connective tissue which is highly innervated and vascularized. The spinal dura mater, a tube which is pierced by the roots of the spinal nerves, extends from the foramen magnum to the second sacral segment. The spinal dura mater is separated from the wall of the spinal canal by the epidural space which contains adipose tissue, the venous plexus and cerebrospinal fluid. The spinal dura mater is also highly vascularized and innervated. For a detailed description of this innervation see Barr and Kiernan.[104] Suffice it to say here that the cranial dura mater and the spinal dura mater have a large sensory innervation so that distortions in the dura are rapidly transmitted throughout the central nervous system and, to a lesser extent, to the peripheral nervous system.

Normal Movement of the Dural Membrane System

Movements of the head and spinal column cause a physiologic change in the shape of the hind brain and the cord.[105] This change in shape is due to the plastic adaptation of the nervous tissue as the spinal column changes length and shape with normal movement. The dura folds and unfolds in an accordion-like manner between the vertebrae, allowing free movement of the nervous tissue. If soft tissue restrictions or bony abnormalities prevent

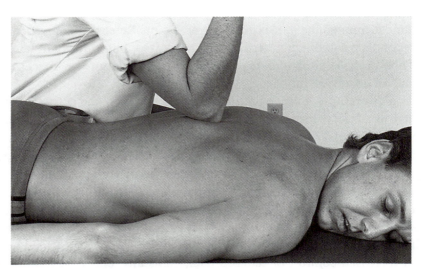

Figure 137A.

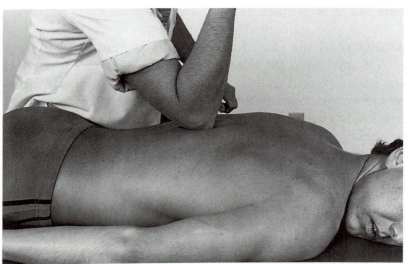

Figure 137B.

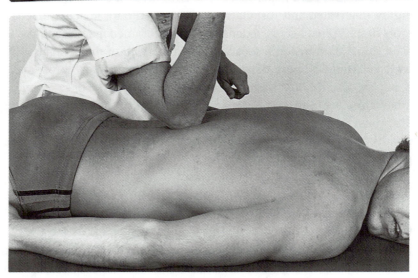

Figure 137C.

Figure 137. Long Stroke Strumming using the elbow. Note the progression of the stroke in pictures A through E.

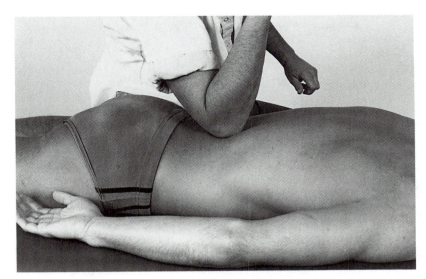

Figure 137D.

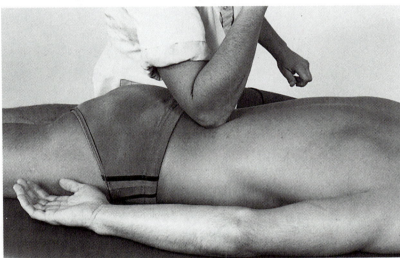

Figure 137E.

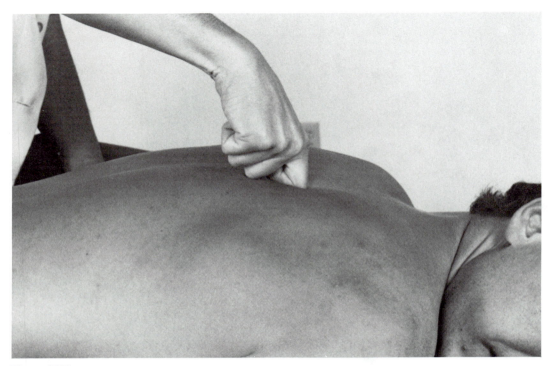

Figure 138A.

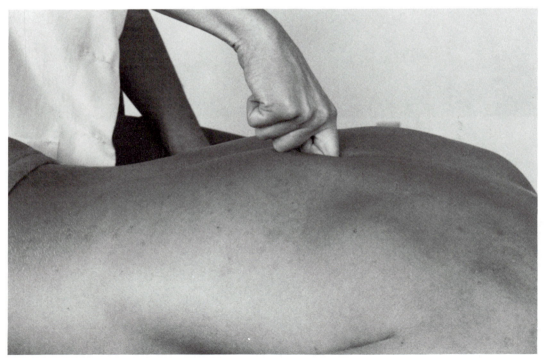

Figure 138B.

Figure 138. Long Stroke Strumming using a knuckle. Note the progression of the stroke in pictures A through D.

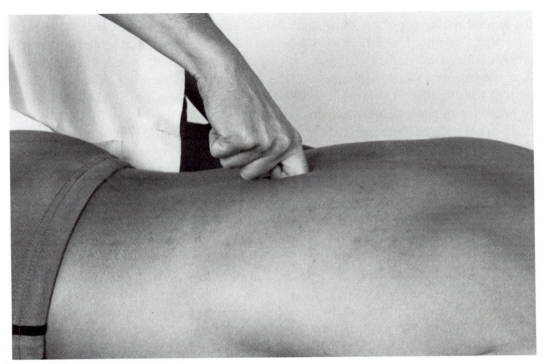

Figure 138C.

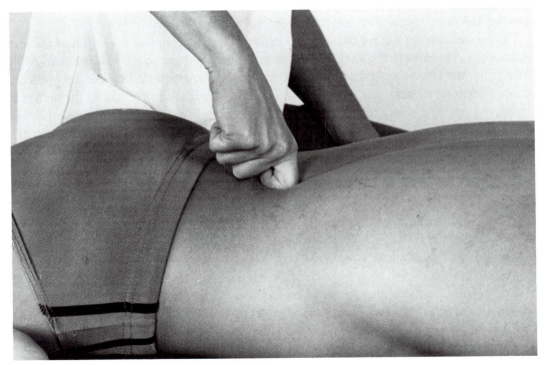

Figure 138D.

the normal movement of the dural tube, normal movement of the nervous tissue is also prevented. In contrast, a flexible dural tube can allow significant bony abnormalities to be present without nerve root impingement and can even accommodate a frankly ruptured disc without neurologic impingement. Therefore, minimal neurologic changes can be present with significant bony abnormalities and significant neurologic abnormalities can be present with minimal bony changes.

There is a significant difference in the mobility of the anterior and posterior surfaces of the cervical and lumbar dura. This is reflected in the different anatomical arrangements of the dura. The dorsal dura, an inelastic membrane, moves by unfolding of the accordion-like folds, while the ventral dura is attached to the posterior surfaces of the vertebral bodies and is held immobile by the nerve roots.[106-108]

When the head is rotated, the cervical canal narrows as the atlas, along with the dura mater, is rotated laterally. The lumen is made smaller by the folds of the dura in much the same way a camera lens is made smaller by the closing of the diaphragm.[105] Thus, if the dura is tight, even a minimal disc protrusion or bony abnormality will give rise to pain and dysfunction.[109]

In normal subjects, forward flexion of the head increases dural tension.[109] As the subject touches the chin to the chest to reach the end range of forward flexion, the dura is placed under greater tension. The dorsal portion of the dura between the occipital bone and the sacrum is 0.5 cm longer than the ventral portion.[105] Using cadavers, Brieg demonstrated that forward flexion of the cervical spine with the trunk held erect stretched the pia mater and ultimately transmitted the resulting tension to the lumbosacral nerve roots and to the sacral cone.[107] Hyperextension of the head shortened the entire dural tube allowing the dura, spinal cord and nerve roots to slacken.[107]

When the anterior surface of the dura relaxes, it forms accordion-like folds at the level of the discs. This allows the anterior dura to protrude slightly into the spinal canal. At the same time, the lateral and posterior surfaces of the dura which lie between the vertebral arches fold and protrude into the spinal canal. Since the dura is attached to the arches by connective tissue, it does not move freely within the canal.[105] Thus, during forward flexion of the head, the cervical nerve roots are displaced upward in the neural foramina. This increases the angle between the nerve roots and the dura,[110] and potentially causes nerve root compression if the foramina is narrowed or if the dura is abnormally tight. The greatest potential for shortening and elongating of the dural tube lies in the posterior part of the cervical vertebral canal.

Lateral flexion of the head causes folding of the dura on the concavity and smoothing or stretching on the convexity. There is potential for nerve root compression on the convex side as the nerve root is displaced upward and on the concave side as the vertebrae approximate.

Axial folding of the dura is present in the atlanto-occipital junction, in the lower cervical region and in the lower thoracic region with the erect posture. The axial dural folds deepen between the atlas and occiput with head rotation. The folds become slightly oblique with this rotation. The greater the amount of rotation, the further distally the effect is observed on the dura.[105]

In the lumbar region, lordosis and kyphosis produce similar movement of the dura. In maximum kyphosis, Brieg found that the posterior portion of the dural tube was elongated 2.2mm,[105] while Charnley determined that the lumbar spine varied 5mm between extreme flexion and extension.[108] If this movement is distributed over the whole length of the lumbar vertebrae, then each extradural root has to accommodate a very small amount of movement. When a patient is asked to perform a pelvic tilt exercise, elongation and stretching of the posterior portion of the dural tube occurs. If the patient is also asked to lift the head, touching chin to chest, the dural tube is placed on maximum stretch, transmitting tension from the sacrum to the occiput and from the occiput to the sacrum.

Pain as an Indicator of Dural Tube Restriction

Pain from the dura mater does not follow the dermatomes. Thus, a lesion in the cervical region can cause pain radiation from the mid-neck down to the scapulae, to the temple and forehead and behind both eyes. This lesion is reflected in the distribution of twelve dermatomes.[111] This wide distribution of pain is due to the innervation of the dura mater by the sinuvertebral nerves along three separate routes. Only the ventral aspect of the dura is innervated.[112] For a detailed discussion of the pain structures within the neural canal, see Massey.[113] Irrespective of where the dura mater is restricted, dural pain is provoked by coughing and in this manner mimics a ruptured intervertebral disc.

Testing for Dural Tube Restriction

Individuals with low postural tone often assume a modified fetal position when upright. Maitland's Slump Test[26] uses this position to test for dural tube restrictions. Overpressure is placed on the spine once a fully rounded position is assumed (Figure 139).

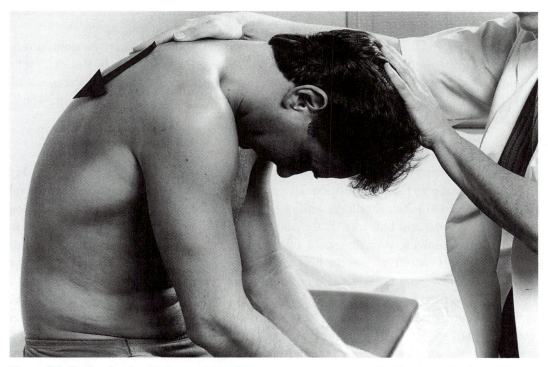

Figure 139. Testing for dural tube restriction by overpressure on your patient's rounded spine.

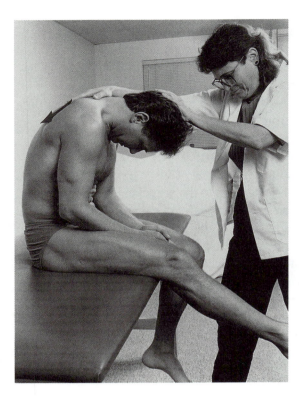

Figure 140. Increasing stretch of the dural tube by extending one knee.

Stretching of the dural tube is increased by having the patient extend one knee while dorsiflexing the foot (Figure 140). Pain would indicate dural tube restrictions.[113]

Straight leg raising tests dural mobility from the fourth lumbar vertebra downward.[26,106,111] Dural tube restrictions are assumed to be present when neck flexion results in low back pain and when pain in the low back during straight leg raising increases with neck flexion. Cyriax and Maitland advocate treating these restrictions with spinal manipulation. Myofascial Release techniques are described below.

Releasing the Dural Tube–One Person Technique

Ask your patient to lie on his side with his head slightly forward flexed and with hip and knees flexed into the fetal position. Use a pillow to maintain his head in neutral lateral flexion (Figure 141). You should be sitting on a stool next to the plinth midway between your patient's head and buttocks. Place one hand on his occiput, cupping the occiput in your palm and allowing your fingers to extend lightly on the back of his head. Place your other hand on his sacrum so that the heel of your hand is at the top of the sacrum and your fingers extend downward over the body of the sacrum (Figures 142 and 143).

Gently push the head upward and forward while pushing the sacrum downward and forward (Figure 144). Hold until a release is felt and proceed as you would for any other release or until spontaneous movement begins. If spontaneous movement begins, follow it keeping a slight amount of drag on the movement so you can feel any hesitations or skips. When no further releases are felt or when the spontaneous movement ceases, again push forward gently on the occiput and sacrum and then pull back gently (Figure 145). Hold this position until a release occurs, spontaneous motion begins or a rocking motion with a

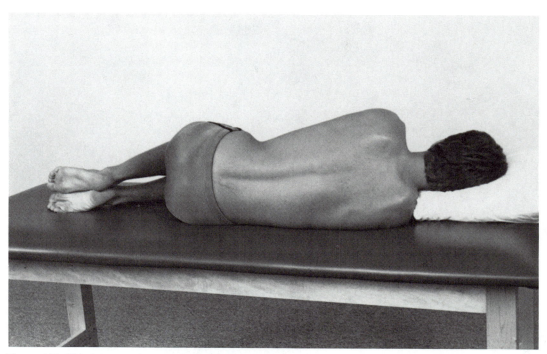

Figure 141. Side-lying position for Releasing the Dural Tube.

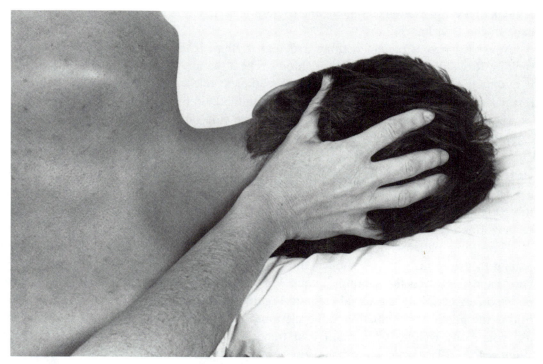

Figure 142. Hand position on the head for Releasing the Dural Tube. The base of the occiput is cradled in the palm of your hand while your fingers lay gently on the back of the head.

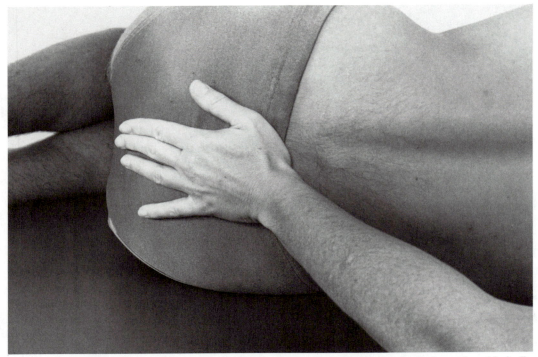

Figure 143. Hand position on the sacrum for Releasing the Dural Tube. The heel of your hand is in firm contact with the sacrum, while your fingers are in firm but light contact with the buttocks.

regular rhythm is established. Once the rhythm is regular, the release is complete and you can remove your hands.

Never leave your patient with an irregular rhythm. If the sacrum and occiput are not rocking forward and backward in synchrony, repeat the above procedure until the rocking is symmetrical. If there were previously incomplete releases in other parts of the body, repeat them when you have completed Releasing the Dural Tube.

If you have a patient who is unable to assume side-lying comfortably, the dural tube can be released with the person prone (Figure 146) or sitting (Figure 147).

Releasing the Dural Tube–Two Person Technique

The two person technique for Releasing the Dural Tube can focus entirely on the dural tube (Figure 148), or a Pelvic Floor Release and a Thoracic Inlet Release (Figure 149) can be performed at the same time, depending upon the skills of the therapists.

Have your patient lying supine in the hook-lying position (Figure 150). Ask your patient to lift up his hips so you can slip your hand between his legs (Figure 151). Place your hand firmly on the sacrum (Figure 152), hooking your fingers over the rim of the pelvis on either side of the spinal column (Figures 153 and 154). As your patient lowers his hips to the plinth, apply traction to the sacrum. Rest on your forearm and lean backward to use your body weight to maintain your traction while your patient straightens his legs (Figure 155). Place your other hand just above your patient's pubis symphysis in proper position for a Pelvic Floor Release (Figure 156).

While the above is happening the therapist who is at the patient's head should be applying cervical traction (see Figures 62-65). Any of the previously described variations

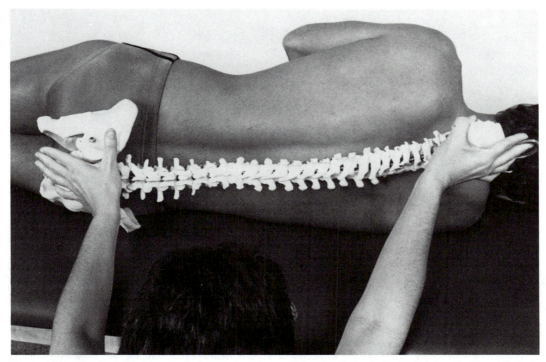

Figure 144A. Hand positions on a skeleton placed over the patient's body for Releasing the Dural Tube in the side-lying position.

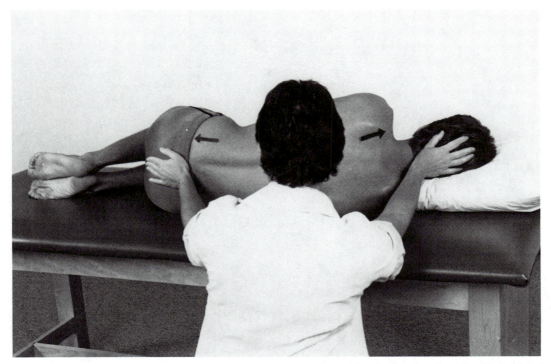

Figure 144B. Apply the initial stretch of the dural tube by gently pushing the head and sacrum forward and then following the inherent tissue motion.

Figure 144. Releasing the Dural Tube in the side-lying position.

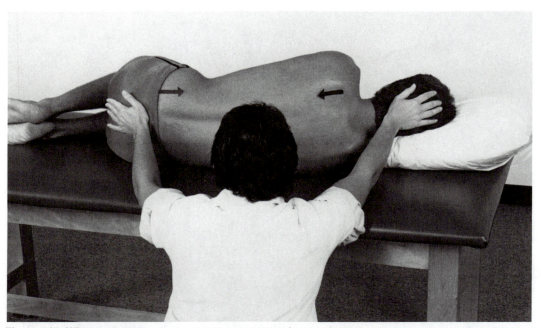

Figure 145. When spontaneous movement ceases or when no further releases occur, push the occiput and sacrum forward at the same time, then pull both back into extension. Follow any spontaneous movement or wait until all releases are complete. A symmetrical rocking forward and backward signals completion of the release.

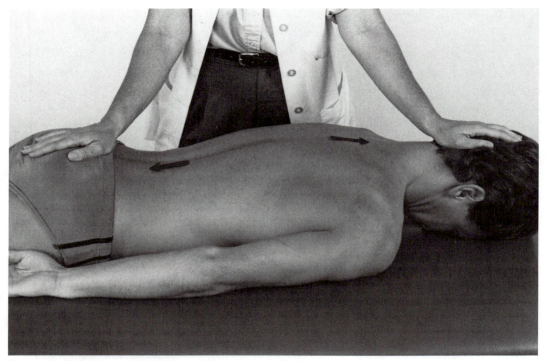

Figure 146. Releasing the Dural Tube with the patient prone.

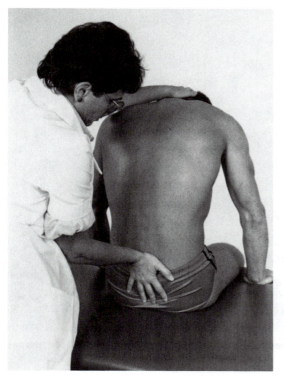

Figure 147. Releasing the Dural Tube with the patient sitting.

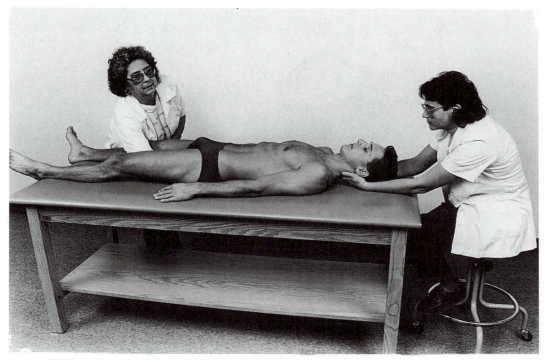

Figure 148. Two person technique for Releasing the Dural Tube.

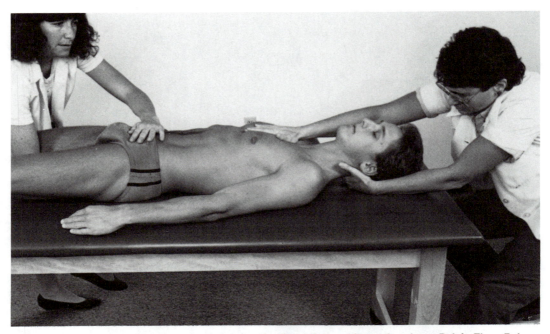

Figure 149. Two person technique for Releasing the Dural Tube while performing a Pelvic Floor Release and a Thoracic Inlet Release.

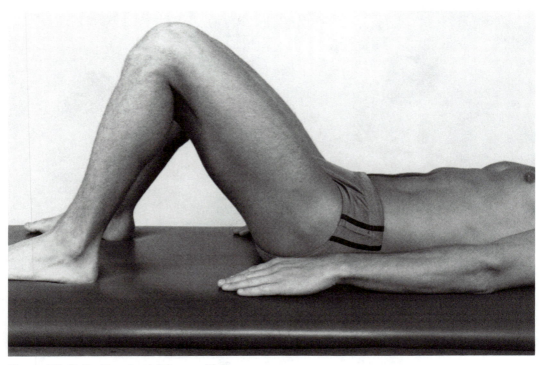

Figure 150. Patient in a hook-lying position.

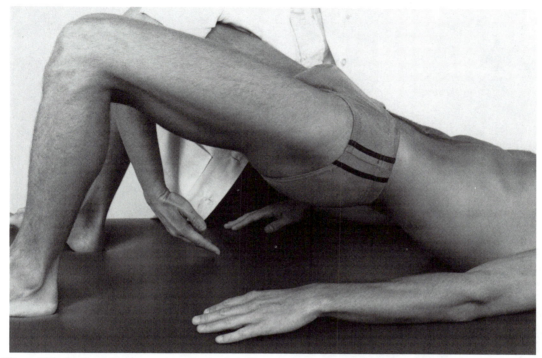

Figure 151. As the patient assumes the body bridge position, the therapist reaches between his legs to place a hand on his sacrum.

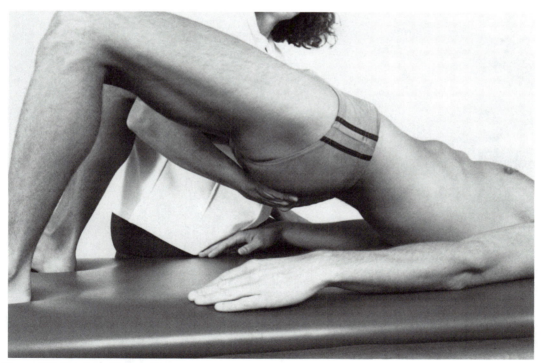

Figure 152. Hand position on the sacrum.

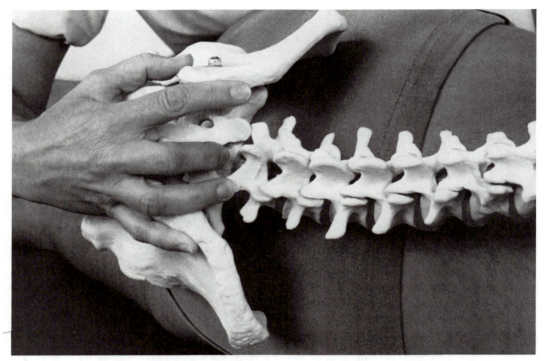

Figure 153. Hand position on a skeleton showing the therapist's fingers gripping the top of the sacrum.

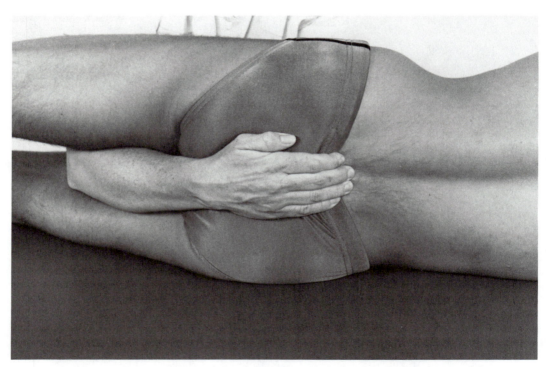

Figure 154. Hand position on the model showing the therapist's fingers gripping the top of the sacrum.

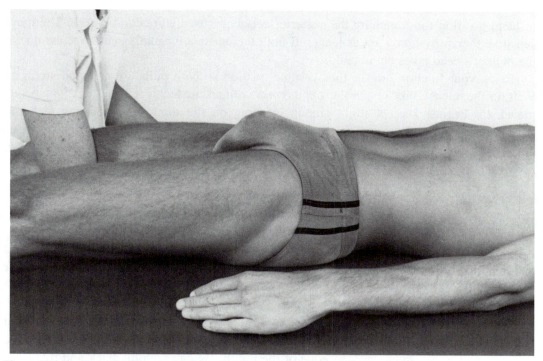

Figure 155. As the patient lowers his hips, the therapist applies traction to the sacrum.

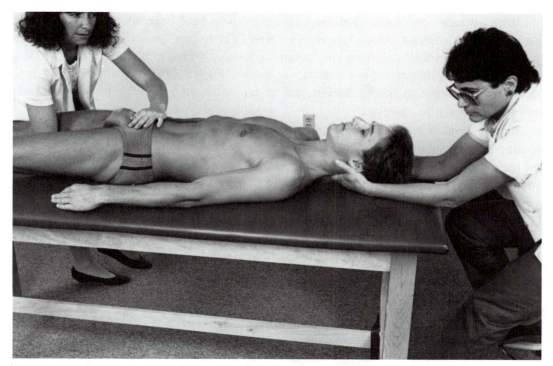

Figure 156. Lightly compressing the lower abdomen while applying traction to the sacrum and the head and neck.

of hand position for stretching the posterior cervical musculature can be used. The more sensitive therapist should act as leader. If both therapists are equally sensitive, the one at the patient's head takes command.

Relax your traction briefly, then resume traction so both pulls are of equal strength. Wait for the release, take up the slack and repeat until an end feel is reached. If spontaneous movement begins, keep a slight amount of drag on the motion so you can feel any hesitations or skips. When all is quiet, apply equal traction again. If no further releases occur, compress the spine and follow any spontaneous motion until an end feel is reached. A symmetrical rocking forward and backward indicates full release of the dural tube.

Treatment in Three Dimensions

Up to this point all of your treatments have been in two dimensions with your patient either supine or prone on the plinth. The third dimension of movement is rotation. In order to also treat the rotation movement dysfunction, your patient must be in free space either sitting or standing.

I prefer to have my patient sitting on a plinth to allow me to maintain a mechanical advantage and to control his position in space. With my patient seated, he can hyperextend his head and/or his spine over the edge of the plinth. He can arch his back and rotate his trunk with or without lateral flexion while sitting or semi-reclined. His head can rotate and flex in the opposite direction from his trunk. His scapulae can protract and retract in combination with any of his trunk and head movements.

With all other Myofascial Release techniques there have been specific starting hand placements. In contrast, when Treating in Three Dimensions, you must rely entirely on your intuition and feedback from your patient to tell you where to place your hands. Most often I place my hands on my patient's scapulae (Figure 157) or on the top of both shoulders and begin to follow the inherent tissue motion and then the more gross body movements when they begin.

If my patient extends one arm, I may place traction on it (Figure 158) or concentrate on placing drag on the trunk movement. If my patient makes a fist, I will push back against his hand compressing his joints (Figure 159). I may perform a Trigger Point Release while stretching a muscle in three dimensions (Figure 160).

You must respond to the feedback from your patient and not anticipate which direction he might move next. Since your patient is in free space and not firmly supported by the plinth, you have lost your margin of safety. If you move in the wrong direction you may lose control of your patient, causing either or both of you to lose your balance. As you both move in three dimensions, the position in which your patient was injured is more easily reproduced. When this happens, your patient may experience an emotional release or a physically facilitated abreaction.[15,16,103]

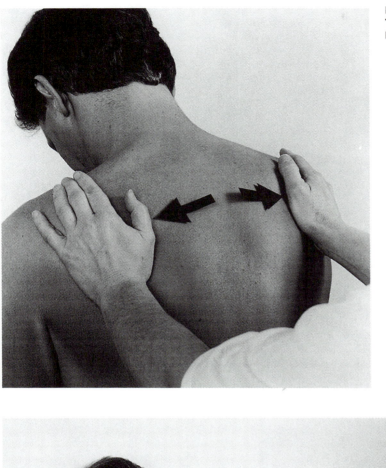

Figure 157. Treatment in Three Dimensions with hands on the scapulae.

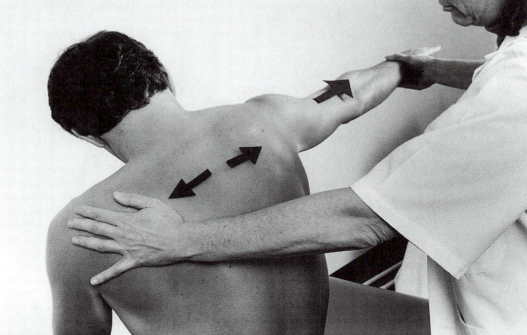

Figure 158. Tractioning the arm in response to a reaching motion.

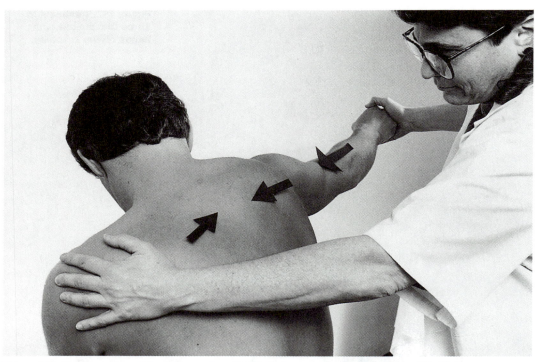

Figure 159. Compression of the upper extremity joints in response to clenching of the fist.

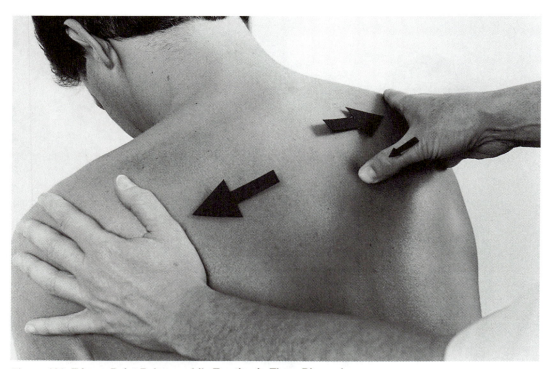

Figure 160. Trigger Point Release while Treating in Three Dimensions.

The Initial Assessment

When planning to use Myofascial Release to treat a patient, a postural assessment must be performed in addition to your regular assessment for a given diagnosis. As usual you must be alert to signs and symptoms that do not correspond to the typical picture presented by that complaint or diagnosis.[114] Assessment is an on-going process. Treatment is modified at each visit in response to your assessment.

Myofascial Release improves postural symmetry. Your initial postural assessment establishes the baseline from which you document change in your clinical notes, in your reports and in discussions with your patients. The postural assessment allows you to monitor change and to determine whether the change is toward symmetry.

Frequently patients cannot detect their initial postural changes. These changes may be so slight as to be not readily noticeable to the untrained eye. Comparing your patient's initial posture with his post-treatment posture will assist him in seeing the changes before he can feel them.

As posture changes, the central nervous system must accept the new sensation before the change can become permanent. There is a conflict between the initial posture which is perceived as "normal" and the improved alignment which is perceived as abnormal. The transitional alignment may, in fact, be less stable than the old alignment. Both the conflict and the temporarily decreased stability may cause increased discomfort or pain. When this happens your patient may become discouraged and want to terminate treatment if you have not forewarned him this would happen. If this happens, showing the improved symmetry to your patient may convince him of the efficacy of the treatment and that, as his body adjusts, he will feel better.

The written assessment may be confusing to your patient. Therefore, for both my benefit and my patient's, I always take photographs at the first visit and periodically thereafter. All four postural views are taken with the patient wearing minimal clothing. These photographs and the negatives are kept in the patient's file. The photographs are mounted, dated and labeled whether pre- or post-treatment.

Quantifying a postural assessment is difficult since you do not want to be standing close to your patient with goniometer, plumb bob and ruler in hand. Once you have measured enough to calibrate your eye, estimates with periodic measurements should be sufficient. Standard range of motion measurements should also be part of the overall assessment. The Assessment Forms which follow give the broad outline of the evaluation process that I use. Depending upon the patient's initial complaint and the complexity of his problem, more or less detail may be required. If you choose to use the following forms, be sure to indicate the degree of deviation; for example, when one shoulder is higher than the other.

One advantage of using assessment forms is that, at a minimum, all of the items on them are assessed periodically. That way, the same items can be noted and change can be quantified. All therapists know well the frustration of sitting down to write a report and finding inconsistent use of specific measures. My frustration is kept to a minimum by the use of these forms. I also use flow charts composed on the computer to speed up writing progress letters and to facilitate following change.

After each re-evaluation, the latest changes are entered on a flow chart; when the flow chart is filled, it is printed and placed in the patient's chart, which is then flagged for a progress letter. A copy of the flow chart is included in the progress letter. This accomplishes two goals. First, the referring doctor receives periodic reports on my letterhead documenting progress of his/her patient. Second, the physician is reminded of the use and benefits of Myofascial Release.

When progress notes are requested by an insurance company before authorizing payment of your bill, this additional documentation will attest to the validity of your treatment and provide quantification of change. Justification of recertification for Medicare is provided in the same way.

For the first part of the initial visit, I take the patient's history in as much detail as the patient feels is necessary. Most of the time, my patient will tell me about his most recent injury and then tell me of other injuries which he thinks contribute to his current problem. In addition to giving my patient a chance to vent any unresolved emotional issues, I gain valuable insight into how my patient views his body and his control over his body. As part of the history I ask my patient to tell me about all surgeries, fractures, scars and other injuries, e.g. strains or sprains going back to childhood. Asking about current medications being taken for any reason will elicit more information than the patient initially volunteers. Occasionally, I will obtain information which my patient has not given his regular physician and which the physician needs for proper medical diagnosis and management of a problem.

If the most recent injury was due to an accident, the history may be an important aid in determining which joints may have been tractioned, compressed or pushed beyond their physiologic range. Initial treatment is directed toward these joints until the myofascial feedback begins to guide the treatment.

The history is placed at the back of the chart and I usually do not look at it again until I am ready to dictate a progress note or discharge letter. The same is true for any notes that I may take. Why bother to listen to the patient's story then? I listen for the very simple reason that the patient needs to tell it and the telling allows a rapport to begin to develop between us. Usually while the story ("I was in a car accident") is being told, I am attempting to extract facts such as "I was thrown to the left" or "My head hit the roof." The reality is that my postural assessment is more important than the patient's story in my decision about where to begin treatment. However, should treatment evolve into a physically facilitated abreaction, this background information can help me anticipate what types of physical movement may occur.[15]

The second part of the initial visit is the postural assessment. It is performed as a strictly hands-off visual inspection. I take photographs at the beginning of the assessment when the patient is holding to his best posture. I then note during the assessment whether the posture changes as the patient relaxes. The major change that is likely to occur is usually in trunk rotation. I dictate this part of the evaluation and mark the assessment forms later. Dictation serves three purposes. First, it is faster for me than marking the forms. Second, a secretary can listen to the dictation, mark the forms for me and add in any additional comments that I made at the time. Third, during dictation the patient's posture is called to his attention by hearing the various landmarks from which I monitor change. When the patient later looks in the mirror, he also sees change and progress. This helps make the patient more of a participant and less of a subject. Many times, a patient will come in eager to report a new change in posture and resulting physical sensation since the last visit, almost in a game of "I saw it first!"

The postural assessment as listed on the forms is quite straightforward. Ask your patient to stand with his back to a wall and his feet several inches away from the wall without being very specific as to how far away. The patient with balance problems, spatial orientation problems, or body image problems will be closer to the wall and may even lean against it. Without being judgmental, ask him to move away from the wall and make note of this behavior. Later, you will be able to decide why your patient stood this way. He may merely have misunderstood your directions.

Always have your patient face you first so that nonverbally you tell your patient that you will never talk behind his back. Ask your patient to focus on a spot which keeps his eyes level and parallel to the floor. I am always seated during the postural assessment so I ask my patients to look at a spot over my head. I prefer to do the postural assessment with patients not wearing glasses. Removing the glasses allows me to see their eyes clearly. It also allows me to detect balance disturbances that are being compensated by vision. If removing the glasses is not possible because taking them off is too stressful in terms of focus or balance disturbance, then I ask my patient to remove his glasses only until I have completed the facial part of the assessment. Before beginning to dictate, I also ask patients to push their hair away from their ears and away from the back of their necks. You do not want a patient to hold his hair with a hand, since this alone changes posture.

At the completion of the postural assessment, if the patient has not been standing with his feet parallel, but with his trunk rotated, I ask him to stand with his feet parallel while facing me. I always stand close to the patient when I ask this because many patients lose their balance when asked to stand this way. If standing with feet parallel does not cause a balance loss, then I can move away and visually inspect again. By asking that the feet be parallel, any trunk rotation will be exaggerated and confirmed. Do not ask a patient to hold this position for long because he will feel uncomfortable and may become irritable. This is an energy-expensive posture to maintain. Specifying a particular stance can be perceived as a criticism of his posture either consciously or subconsciously.

Next assess skin mobility with your patient standing. You may want to re-assess skin mobility while your patient is sitting or lying down. Scars are always palpated for restriction during this part of the assessment.

Spinal movement and sacro-iliac movement should be assessed in the standing position.[115] First, assess visually before palpating the movement. The most important aspect is the quality of movement. Symmetry and asymmetry of movement need to be noted. Generally, symmetry allows the most energy-efficient movement patterns or the best compensation available for limited movement. Rarely, if ever, is a pathological condition symmetrical. The patient will often perform a motion without movement occurring at the proper spinal segments. Much important information is lost if only quantity of movement is noted. Immobility and hypermobility must be localized to vertebral level. Most therapists are accustomed to doing this in the lumbar area but neglect doing it in the thoracic and cervical areas. Spinal and sacro-iliac movement should be reassessed with the patient sitting to identify any effect of tight leg musculature on the pelvis. Thus, the assessment process is a systematic approach that will identify restricted myofascial structures and guide your initial treatment approach.

The myofascial restrictions identified in this manner are only the most obvious and most superficial in terms of effect on the entire body. Ultimately, the key restricted structures will not be those identified during the initial assessment. According to the onion metaphor, the most superficial restrictions are treated first to allow access to the deeper restrictions. As each layer is treated, deeper or more fundamental restrictions are located and become accessible to the therapist's hands. Treatment continues until "the core of the onion" is reached and treated.

Keep in mind that the body is a kinetic chain. A change in the ability to move any part of the body affects the ability to move every other part of the body. Postural malalignment in any part of the body causes postural malalignment throughout the entire body.

The most dramatic illustration of the effects of one part of the body on all other parts is the patient with a flaccid paralysis due to peripheral nerve injury caused by disease or an accident. The entire body must adjust to the passive malposition. In contrast, spastic paralysis dynamically causes malposition. While the presence of both of these problems makes myofascial treatment less efficient and beneficial, neither is a contraindication to myofascial stretching. In fact, myofascial stretching is the safest method of stretching in the presence of flaccid paralysis because the feedback from the patient's body will prevent over-stretching and will thus allow protective tightness to remain.

Once the standing and sitting evaluations are completed, the supine evaluation is performed. Actual measurement of leg length must be performed from whatever reproducible landmark with which you are comfortable. Remember that many leg length discrepancies are due to asymmetry of the pelvis. A leg length discrepancy reaching back into childhood can still be changed with myofascial stretching. Long-standing scoliosis which is not due to vertebral wedging can be reduced by stretching and balancing the soft tissues. Anatomic changes cannot be overcome, but the soft tissue response to them may be modified.

Conclusion

This manual is only an introduction to the concept of Myofascial Release. The key to Myofascial Release is the sensitivity of your hands. The only way to develop and refine this skill is to place your hands on as many different people as possible to learn the feel of the soft tissues and their inherent motion. Next, you must learn to trust what you are feeling through your hands and respond to those feelings. Allow your patients to lead you and direct their treatment. Above all, become comfortable with yourself, be relaxed, and allow yourself to explore alternative ways to relate to your patients and respond to their needs. Your use of Myofascial Release is limited only by the sensitivity of your hands and your creativity in responding to feedback.

IV

Additional Resources

Assessment Forms

Part I. Postural Assessment

STANDING

I. Facing Forward

Head Tilt
- neutral
- left
- right

Head Rotation
- neutral
- left
- right

Facial Crease
- equal
- deeper left
- deeper right

Eyes
- level
- left higher
- right higher
- equal size
- left bigger
- right bigger

Mouth
- symmetrical
- left longer
- right longer

- not pulled
- pulled left
- pulled right
- level
- left elevated
- right elevated

Nose
- midline
- deviated left
- deviated right

Ears
- level
- left elevated
- right elevated
- neutral
- left externally rotated
- right externally rotated
- left internally rotated
- right internally rotated

Neck
- equal length
- left longer
- right longer

Shoulders
- equal length
- left longer
- right longer
- level
- left elevated
- right elevated
- neutral
- left protracted
- right protracted
- left retracted
- right retracted

Arms
- neutral
- left external rotation
- right external rotation
- left internal rotation
- right internal rotation
- equal length
- left longer
- right longer
- equal abduction
- left greater abduction
- right greater abduction

Trunk
neutral
shifted left
shifted right
sides equal length
  left longer
  right longer
equal creases
  left higher
  right higher
  left longer
  right longer
neutral rotation
  rotated left
  rotated right
Pelvis
level
left higher
right higher
neutral
left retracted
right retracted
left protracted
right protracted
Thighs
neutral
left external rotation
right external rotation
left internal rotation
right internal rotation
Knees
level
left higher
right higher
equal
left recurvatum
right recurvatum
left flexed
right flexed
Lower Leg
neutral
left varus
right varus
left valgus
right valgus

Foot
neutral left
neutral right
pronated left
pronated right
inverted left
inverted right
Forefoot
neutral left
neutral right
left varus
right varus
left valgus
right valgus
Weight Bearing
equal
greater left
greater right

II. Facing Right
Head
neutral
forward
hyperextended
Ear
over acromium
forward of acromium
behind acromium
Shoulder
over hip
forward of hip
behind hip
neutral
protracted
retracted
Hip
over middle of knee
  joint
forward of knee joint
behind knee joint
neutral
protracted
retracted
over malleolus

forward of malleolus
behind malleolus
Knee
neutral
flexed
recurvatum
over malleolus
forward of malleolus
behind malleolus
Cervical Lordosis
WNL
exaggerated
flattened
equals lumbar lordosis
greater than lumbar
  lordosis
less than lumbar
  lordosis
Thoracic Kyphosis
WNL
exaggerated
flattened
Lumbar Lordosis
WNL
exaggerated
flattened

III. Facing Backwards
Head Tilt
neutral
left
right
Head Rotation
neutral
left
right
Ears
level
left elevated
right elevated
neutral
left externally rotated
right externally
  rotated

left internally rotated
right internally
   rotated
Neck
   equal length
   left longer
   right longer
Shoulders
   equal length
   left longer
   right longer
   level
   left elevated
   right elevated
   neutral
   left protracted
   right protracted
   left retracted
   right retracted
Arms
   neutral
   left external rotation
   right external rotation
   left internal rotation
   right internal rotation
   equal length
   left longer
   right longer
   equal abduction
   left greater
      abduction
   right greater
      abduction
Trunk
   neutral
   shifted left
   shifted right
   sides equal length
      left longer
      right longer
   equal creases
      left higher
      right higher
      left longer
      right longer

neutral rotation
   rotated left
   rotated right
Pelvis
   level
   left higher
   right higher
   neutral
   left retracted
   right retracted
   left protracted
   right protracted
Thighs
   neutral
   left external rotation
   right external rotation
   left internal rotation
   right internal rotation
Knees
   level
   left higher
   right higher
   equal
   left recurvatum
   right recurvatum
   left flexed
   right flexed
Lower Leg
   neutral
   left varus
   right varus
   left valgus
   right valgus
Foot
   neutral left
   neutral right
   pronated left
   pronated right
   inverted left
   inverted right
Weight Bearing
   equal
   greater left
   greater right

IV. Facing Left
   Head
      neutral
      forward head
      hyperextended
   Ear
      over acromium
      forward of acromium
      behind acromium
   Shoulder
      over hip
      forward of hip
      behind hip
      neutral
      protracted
      retracted
   Hip
      over middle of knee
         joint
      forward of knee joint
      behind knee joint
      neutral
      protracted
      retracted
      over malleolus
      forward of malleolus
      behind malleolus
   Knee
      neutral
      flexed
      recurvatum
      over malleolus
      forward of malleolus
      behind malleolus
   Cervical Lordosis
      WNL
      exaggerated
      flattened
      equals lumbar lordosis
      greater than lumbar
         lordosis
      less than lumbar
         lordosis

Thoracic Kyphosis
WNL
exaggerated
flattened
Lumbar Lordosis
WNL
exaggerated
flattened

SITTING

I. Facing Forward
Head Tilt
neutral
left
right
Head Rotation
neutral
left
right
Facial Crease
equal
deeper left
deeper right
Eyes
level
left higher
right higher
equal size
left bigger
right bigger
Mouth
symmetrical
left longer
right longer
not pulled
pulled left
pulled right
level
left elevated
right elevated
Nose
midline
deviated left
deviated right

Ears
level
left elevated
right elevated
neutral
left externally rotated
right externally
rotated
left internally rotated
right internally
rotated
Neck
equal length
left longer
right longer
Shoulders
equal length
left longer
right longer
level
left elevated
right elevated
neutral
left protracted
right protracted
left retracted
right retracted
Arms
neutral
left external rotation
right external rotation
left internal rotation
right internal rotation
equal length
left longer
right longer
equal abduction
left greater
abduction
right greater
abduction
Trunk
neutral
shifted left
shifted right

sides equal length
left longer
right longer
equal creases
left higher
right higher
left longer
right longer
neutral rotation
rotated left
rotated right

II. Facing Right
Head
neutral
forward
hyperextended
Ear
over acromium
forward of acromium
behind acromium
Shoulder
over hip
forward of hip
behind hip
neutral
protracted
retracted
Pelvis
level
left higher
right higher
neutral
left retracted
right retracted
left protracted
right protracted
Cervical Lordosis
WNL
exaggerated
flattened
equals lumbar lordosis
greater than lumbar
lordosis

less than lumbar
lordosis
Thoracic Kyphosis
WNL
exaggerated
flattened
Lumbar Lordosis
WNL
exaggerated
flattened

III. Facing Backwards
Head Tilt
neutral
left
right
Head Rotation
neutral
left
right
Ears
level
left elevated
right elevated
neutral
left externally rotated
right externally
rotated
left internally rotated
right internally
rotated
Neck
equal length
left longer
right longer
Shoulders
equal length
left longer
right longer
level

left elevated
right elevated
neutral
left protracted
right protracted
left retracted
right retracted
Arms
neutral
left external rotation
right external rotation
left internal rotation
right internal rotation
equal length
left longer
right longer
equal abduction
left greater
abduction
right greater
abduction
Trunk
neutral
shifted left
shifted right
sides equal length
left longer
right longer
equal creases
left higher
right higher
left longer
right longer
neutral rotation
rotated left
rotated right
Pelvis
level
left higher
right higher
neutral

left retracted
right retracted
left protracted
right protracted

IV. Facing Left
Head
neutral
forward
hyperextended
Ear
over acromium
forward of acromium
behind acromium
Shoulder
over hip
forward of hip
behind hip
neutral
protracted
retracted
Cervical Lordosis
WNL
exaggerated
flattened
equals lumbar lordosis
greater than lumbar
lordosis
less than lumbar
lordosis
Thoracic Kyphosis
WNL
exaggerated
flattened
Lumbar Lordosis
WNL
exaggerated
flattened

Part II. Analysis of Movement

STANDING

I. Cervical

Rotation Left
full 3/4 1/2 1/4 1/8 0

Rotation Right
full 3/4 1/2 1/4 1/8 0

Lateral Flexion Left
full 3/4 1/2 1/4 1/8 0

Lateral Flexion Right
full 3/4 1/2 1/4 1/8 0

Hyperextension
full 3/4 1/2 1/4 1/8 0

Forward Flexion
chin touches chest
1 finger 2 3 4 minimal

II. Thoracic and Lumbar

A. Forward Flexion–fingertips to:
 floor
 top of foot
 ankle
 above ankle
 mid calf
 middle of knee
 mid thigh
 hip joints

smooth symmetrical thoracic curve

asymmetrical thoracic curve
 flattened thorax
 sharply angled apex at:
 immobile segments
 hypermobile segments

smooth reversal lumbar lordotic curve
 flattened low back
 immobile segments
 hypermobile segments

B. Left Lateral Flexion–fingertips to:
 floor
 top of foot
 ankle
 above ankle
 mid calf
 middle of knee
 mid thigh
 hip joints

smooth symmetrical thoracic curve

asymmetrical thoracic curve
 flattened
 sharply angled apex at:
 immobile thoracic segments
 hypermobile thoracic segments

smooth lumbar curve right

flat lumbar curve right
 immobile lumbar segments
 hypermobile lumbar segments

C. Right Lateral Flexion–fingertips to:
floor
top of foot
ankle
above ankle
mid calf
middle of knee
mid thigh
hip joints

smooth symmetrical thoracic curve

asymmetrical thoracic curve
flattened
sharply angled apex at:
immobile segments
hypermobile segments

smooth reversal lumbar lordotic curve
flattened low back
immobile segments
hypermobile segments

D. Hyperextension
full 3/4 1/2 1/4 1/8 0
smooth curve
asymmetrical
fulcrum at:
immobile segments
hypermobile segments

E. Legs–Squat Test
both heels on floor to end range
left heel on floor to end range
left heel lifts
right heel on floor to end range
right heel lifts

SITTING

I. Cervical

Rotation Left
full 3/4 1/2 1/4 1/8 0

Rotation Right
full 3/4 1/2 1/4 1/8 0

Lateral Flexion Left
full 3/4 1/2 1/4 1/8 0

Lateral Flexion Right
full 3/4 1/2 1/4 1/8 0

Hyperextension
full 3/4 1/2 1/4 1/8 0

Forward Flexion
chin touches chest
1 finger 2 3 4 minimal

II. Thoracic and Lumbar

A. Forward Flexion
smooth symmetrical thoracic curve

asymmetrical thoracic curve
flattened
sharply angled apex at:
immobile thoracic segments
hypermobile thoracic segments

smooth reversal lumbar lordotic curve
flattened low back
immobile lumbar segments
hypermobile lumbar segments

B. Left Lateral Flexion
smooth symmetrical thoracic curve

asymmetrical thoracic curve
flattened
sharply angled apex at:
immobile thoracic segments
hypermobile thoracic segments

smooth lumbar curve right
flat lumbar curve right
immobile lumbar segments
hypermobile lumbar segments

C. Right Lateral Flexion
smooth symmetrical thoracic curve

asymmetrical thoracic curve
flattened
sharply angled apex at:

immobile thoracic segments
hypermobile thoracic segments

smooth lumbar curve left
  flat lumbar curve left
  immobile lumbar segments
  hypermobile lumbar segments

D. Hyperextension
full 3/4 1/2 1/4 1/8 0
smooth curve
asymmetrical
  fulcrum at:
  immobile segments
  hypermobile segments

Part III. Palpation

STANDING

I. Skin Mobility
Anterior Chest Wall Tightness
  upward
  downward
  left
  right
Anterior Abdominal Wall Tightness
  upward
  downward
  left
  right
Upper Thoracic Tightness
  upward
  downward
  left
  right
Lower Thoracic Tightness
  upward
  downward
  left
  right
Lumbar Tightness
  upward
  downward
  left
  right

II. Anterior Superior Iliac Crests
  equal height
  left higher
  right higher
  left lower
  right lower
  neutral rotation
  left rotated up
  right rotated up
  left rotated down
  right rotated down

III. Posterior Superior Iliac Crests
  equal height
  left higher
  right higher
  left lower
  right lower
  neutral rotation
  left rotated up
  right rotated up
  left rotated down
  right rotated down

SUPINE

I. Skin Mobility
Anterior Chest Wall Tightness
  upward
  downward
  left
  right

Anterior Abdominal Wall Tightness
  upward
  downward
  left
  right

II. Anterior Superior Iliac Crests
equal height
left higher
right higher
left lower
right lower
neutral rotation
left rotated up
right rotated up
left rotated down
right rotated down

III. Pubic Tubercles
equal height
left higher
right higher
left lower
right lower
neutral rotation
left rotated up
right rotated up
left rotated down
right rotated down

IV. Leg Lengths
left medial malleolus higher
right medial malleolus higher
left medial malleolus lower
right medial malleolus lower
measured leg lengths
   left
   right

PRONE

I. Skin Mobility

Upper Thoracic Tightness
upward
downward
left
right
Lower Thoracic Tightness
upward
downward
left
right
Lumbar Tightness
upward
downward
left
right

II. Posterior Superior Iliac Crests
equal height
left higher
right higher
left lower
right lower
neutral rotation
left rotated up
right rotated up
left rotated down
right rotated down

III. Sacral Sulci
equal
left higher
right higher
left lower
right lower

IV. Sacral Tuberous Ligament
equal
left higher
right higher
left lower
right lower

Part IV. Observation

I. Leg Position with Hip and Knee Extended
rotation
    left neutral
    right neutral

Left External Rotation
full 3/4 1/2 1/4 0

Right External Rotation
full 3/4 1/2 1/4 0

Left Internal Rotation
full 3/4 1/2 1/4 0

Right Internal Rotation
full 3/4 1/2 1/4 0

abduction/adduction
left neutral
right neutral
left abduction
right abduction
left adduction
right adduction

II. Gluteal Cleft
midline
deviated left
deviated right

Part V. Range of Motion Measurements

SUPINE

I. Cervical

left
active   passive

right
passive   active

II. Neck
forward flexion
extension
hyperextension
rotation
lateral flexion

UPPER EXTREMITY

left
active   passive

right
passive   active

I. Shoulder
flexion
extension
abduction
horizontal adduction
external rotation
internal rotation

II. Elbow
flexion
extension
supination
pronation

III. Wrist
flexion
extension
dorsiflexion
radial deviation
ulnar deviation

LOWER EXTREMITY

	left			right	
	active	passive		passive	active

I. Hip
flexion
extension
abduction
adduction
external rotation
internal rotation

II. Knee
flexion
extension

III. Ankle
dorsiflexion
plantarflexion
inversion
eversion

Cited References

1. Kegerreis SK: Myofascial therapy and the infomedical model: a rationale for clinician connectedness. Presented at the APTA National Conference: June 15, 1992; Denver, CO.

2. Grodin AJ, Cantu RI: Soft tissue mobilization. In: Basmajian JV, Nyberg R, eds. *Rational Manual Therapies*, Baltimore, MD, Williams and Wilkins, 1993: 199-221.

3. Ward RC: Myofascial release concepts. In: Basmajian JV, Nyberg R, eds. *Rational Manual Therapies*. Baltimore, MD, Williams and Wilkins, 1963: 223-241.

4. Juhan D: *Job's Body*. Barrytown, NY, Station Hill Press, 1987, vii-xxxi.

5. Irby DM: Shifting paradigms of research in medical education. *Academic Medicine* 65:622-623, 1991.

6. Harris JD: History and development of manipulation and mobilization. In: Basmajian JV, Nyberg R, eds. *Rational Manual Therapies*. Baltimore, MD, Williams and Wilkins, 1993, 7-19.

7. Osler W: In discussion: Cannon DS. In: *The Healing Heart*. New York, WW Norton & Co, 1983, 256.

8. Lewis CS: *Miracles*. New York, The Macmillan Co, 1947, 168.

9. Rolf I: *Rolfing: The Integration of Human Structure*. Santa Monica, CA: Dennis Landman Publishing Co; 1977.

10. Kendall FP, McCreary EK: *Muscles Testing and Function*, 3rd ed. Baltimore, MD, Williams and Wilkins, 1983, 11.

11. Cailliet R: *Soft Tissue Pain and Disability*. Philadelphia, FA Davis Company, 1977.

12. Taylor TC: Myofascial release techniques. *Physical Therapy Forum* 23:1-3, June 4, 1986.

13. Montagu, A: *Touching: The Human Significance of the Skin*. New York, Columbia University Press, 1971.

14. Lidell, L: *The Sensual Body: The Ultimate Guide to Body Awareness and Self-fulfilment*. New York, Simon and Schuster, Inc, 1987.

15. Manheim, CJ: Psychological Effects of Manual Therapy. Presented at the APTA National Conference: June 15, 1992; Denver, CO.

16. Manheim CJ, Lavett DK: *Craniosacral Therapy and Somato-Emotional Release: The Self-Healing Body*. Thorofare, NJ, SLACK Inc, 1989.

17. Davis CM: *Patient Practitioner Interaction: An Experiential Manual for Developing the Art of Health Care*. Thorofare, NJ, SLACK Inc, 1989.

18. Swansea, CW: *Mindworks: How to Become a More Creative and Critical Thinker*. Columbia, SC, South Carolina ETV, 1990.

19. Travell JG, Simons DG: *Myofascial Pain and Dysfunction: The Trigger Point Manual*. Baltimore, William & Wilkins, 1983.

20. Upledger JE, Vredevoogd JD: *Craniosacral Therapy*. Seattle WA, Eastland Press, 1983.

21. Garfin SR, Tipton CM, Mubarek, SJ, et al: Role of fascia in maintenance of muscle tension and pressure. *J Appl Physiol, Respiratory, Environmental and Exercise Physiology* 51:317-320, 1981.

22. Tortota, GJ, Anagnostakos, NP: *Principles of Anatomy and Physiology*. 5th ed. New York, Harper & Row, Publishers, 1987.

23. Hollinshead WH: *Functional Anatomy of The Limbs and Back*, 2nd. edition. Philadelphia, W.B. Saunders Company, 1960.

24. Schaeffer JP (ed): *Morris' Human Anatomy*, 11th ed. New York, McGraw-Hill Book Company, Inc. 1953.

25. Hoppenfeld S, Hutton R: *Physical Examination of The Spine and Extremities*. New York, Appleton-Century-Crofts, 1976.

26. Maitland GD: *Vertebral Manipulation*. London, Butterworth & Company, Ltd, 1986.

27. Kemp, ML: *Merlin's Body Balance: A Message of Health*. Santa Barbara, CA, The Campanile Press, 1986.

28. Ebner M: *Connective Tissue Massage: Theory and Therapeutic Application.* Huntington, New York, Robert E. Krieger Publishing Company, 1962.

29. Udolf, R: *Handbook of Hypnosis for Professionals*, 2nd ed. Northvale, NJ, Jason Aronson Inc, 1992.

30. Bonica JJ: Management of myofascial pain syndromes in general practice. *JAMA* 164:732-738, 1957.

31. Campbell SM, Bennett RM: Fibrositis. *Disease A Month* 32:653- 722, 1986a.

32. Campbell SM: Is the tender point concept valid? *Am J Med* 81:3:33-37, 1986b.

33. Eisenberg D, Wright TL: *Encounters with Qi: Exploring Chinese Medicine.* New York, Norton, 1985.

34. Gorrell RL: Musculofascial pain: Treatment by local injection of analgesic drugs. *JAMA* 142:557-561, 1950.

35. Grosshandler S, Stratas NE, Toomey TC, et al: Chronic neck and shoulder pain. Focusing on myofascial origins. *Postgrad Med* 77:149-158, 1985.

36. Jaeger B, Reeves JL: Quantification of changes in myofascial trigger point sensitivity with the pressure algometer following passive stretch. *Pain* 27:203-210, 1986.

37. Reynolds MD: Myofascial trigger points in persistent posttraumatic shoulder pain. *South Med J* 77:1277-1280, 1984.

38. Russell J, Vipraio GA, Morgan WW, et al: Is there a metabolic basis for the fibrositis syndrome? *Am J Med* 81:50-54, 1986.

39. Simons DG: Fibrositis/fibromyalgia: A form of myofascial trigger points? *Am J Med* 81:93-98, 1986.

40. Simons DG: Myofascial pain syndrome due to trigger points. *International Rehabilitation Medicine Association Monograph Series* 1:1-39, 1987.

41. Slocumb JC: Neurological factors in chronic pelvic pain: Trigger points and the abdominal pelvic pain syndrome. *Am J Obstet Gynecol* 536-543, July 1984.

42. Tunks E, Crook J, Norman G, et al: Tender points in fibromyalgia. *Pain* 34:11-19, 1988.

43. Yunus M, Masi AT, Feigenbaum SL, et al: Primary fibromyalgia (fibrositis): Clinical study of 50 patients with matched normal controls. *Semin Arthritis Rheum* 11:151-171, 1981.

44. Inman VT, Saunders JBDM: Referred pain from skeletal structures. *J Nerv Men Dis* 99:660-667, 1944.

45. Bates T, Grunwaldt E: Myofascial pain in childhood. *J Pediatr* 53:198-209, 1958.

46. Berges PU: Myofascial pain syndromes. *Postgrad Med* 53:161-168, 1973.

47. Grosshandler S, Burney R: The myofascial syndrome. *NC Med J* 40:562-565, 1979.

48. Gunn CC, Milbrandt ME: Shoulder pain, cervical spondylosis and acupuncture. *American Journal of Acupuncture* 5:121-128, 1977.

49. Hockaday JM, Whitty CWM: Patterns of referred pain in the normal subject. *Brain* 90:481-496, 1967.

50. Jaeger B: Myofascial referred pain patterns: The role of trigger points. *Journal of The California Dental Association* 13:27-28, 1985.

51. Kellgren JH: A preliminary account of referred pains arising from muscle. *Br Med J* 1:325-327, 1938.

52. Kleier DJ: Referred pain from a myofascial trigger point mimicking pain of endodontic origin. *Journal of Endodontics* 11:408-411, 1985.

53. Lewis T, Kellgren JH: Observations relating to referred pain, visceromotor reflexes and other associated phenomena. *Clin Sci* 1:47-71, 1939.

54. Melzack R, Stillwell DM, Fox EJ: Trigger points and acupuncture points for pain: Correlations and implications. *Pain* 3:3-23, 1977.

55. Pace JB: Commonly overlooked pain syndromes responsive to simple therapy. *Postgrad Med* 58:107-113, 1975.

56. Schwartz RG, Gall NG, Grant AE: Abdominal pain in quadriparesis: Myofascial syndrome as unsuspected cause. *Arch Phys Med Rehabil* 65:44-46, 1984.

57. Simons DG, Travell JG: Myofascial origins of low back pain: I: Principles of diagnosis and treatment. *Postgrad Med* 73:66-77, 1983.

58. Simons, DG, Travell JG: Myofascial origins of low back pain: II: Torso muscles. *Postgrad Med* 73:81-92, 1983.

59. Simons DG, Travell JG: Myofascial origins of low back pain: III: Pelvic and lower extremity muscles. *Postgrad Med* 73:99-108, 1983.

60. Sola AE, Kuitert JH: Myofascial trigger point pain in the neck and shoulder girdle. *Northwest Medicine* 980-984, 1955.

61. Travell JG: Temporomandibular Joint Pain referred from muscles of the head and neck. *J Prosthe Dent* 10:745-763, 1960.

62. Travell JG: Identification of myofascial trigger point syndromes: A case of atypical facial neuralgia. *Arch Phys Med Rehabil* 62:100-106, 1981.

63. Travell JG, Rinzler SH: The myofascial genesis of pain. *Postgrad Med* 11:425-434, 1952.

64. Wyant GM: Chronic pain syndromes and their treatment. The piriformis syndrome. *Canadian Anaesthiology Society Journal* 26:305-308, 1979.

65. Wyant GM: Chronic pain syndromes and their treatment. Trigger Points. *Canadian Anaesthiology Society Journal* 26:216-219, 1979.

66. Butler JH, Folke LEA, Bandt CL: A descriptive survey of signs and symptoms associated with the myofascial pain-dysfunction syndrome. *J Am Den Assoc* 90:635-639, 1975.

67. Fricton JR, Auvinen MD, Dykstra D, et al: Myofascial pain syndrome: Electromyographic changes associated with local twitch response. *Arch Phys Med Rehabil* 66:314-317, 1985.

68. Fricton JR, Kroening R, Haley D, et al: Myofascial pain syndrome of the head and neck: A review of clinical characteristics of 164 patients. *Oral Surgery* 60:615-623, 1985.

69. Lewit K, Simons DG: Myofascial pain: Relief by post-isometric relaxation. *Arch Phys Med Rehabil* 65:452-456, 1984.

70. MacDonald AJR: Abnormally tender muscle regions and associated painful movements. *Pain* 8:197-205, 1980.

71. Coulehan J: Primary fibromyalgia. *Am Fam Physician* 32:170-177, 1985.

72. Leandrim M, Brunetti O, Parodi, CI: Telethermographic findings after transcutaneous electrical nerve stimulation. *Phys Ther* 66:210-213, 1986.

73. Sheon RP: Regional myofascial pain and the fibrositis syndrome (fibromyalgia). *Compr Ther* 12:42-52, 1986.

74. Snyder-Mackler L, Bork C, Bourbon B, et al: Effect of helium-neon laser on musculoskeletal trigger points. *Phys Ther* 66:1087-1090, 1986.

75. Wolfe F: Development of criteria for the diagnosis of fibrositis. *Am J Med* 81:99-104, 1986.

76. Schmalbruch H: Contracture knots in normal and diseased muscle fibres. *Brain* 96:637-640, 1973.

77. Simons DG: Muscle pain syndromes. *Am J Phys Med* Part I 54:289-311, 1975 ; Part II 55:15-42, 1976.

78. Dexter JR, Simons DG: Local twitch response in human muscle evoked by palpation and needle penetration of a trigger point. *Arch Phys Med Rehabil* 62:521, 1981.

79. Kine G, Warfield C: Myofascial pain syndrome. *Hosp Prac* 21:194B-194C,194G-194H, 1986.

80. Dittrich RJ: Low back pain - referred pain from deep somatic structure of the back. *Lancet* 73:63-68, 1953.

81. Defalque RJ: Painful trigger points in surgical scars. *Anesthesia and Analgesia* 61:518-520, 1982.

82. Epstein SE, Gerber LH, Borer JS: Chest wall syndrome. *JAMA* 241:2793-2797, 1979.

83. Rinzler SH, Travell JG: Therapy directed at the somatic component of cardiac pain. *Am Heart J* 35:248-268, 1948.

84. Manheim CJ, Lavett DK: A Myofascial Trigger Point That Causes Gastrointestinal Symptoms. Proceedings of the World Confederation for Physical Therapy, 11th International Conference. Book II. London, 1991.

85. Rubin D: Myofascial trigger point syndromes: An approach to management. *Arch Phys Med Rehabil* 62:107-110, 1981.

86. Ruskin AP: Facial neuralgia with trigger point on finger, one case suggesting a cortically mediated response. *Arch Neurol* 37:672, 1980.

87. Travell JG: A trigger point for hiccup. *J Am Osteopath Assoc* 77:308-312, 1977.

88. Fine PG: Myofascial trigger point pain in children. *J Pediatr* 111:547-548, 1987.

89. Laskin DM: Etiology of the pain-dysfunction syndrome. *J Am Dent Assoc* 79:147-153, 1969.

90. Graff-Radford SB, Jaeger B, Reeves JL: Myofascial pain may present clinically as occipital neuralgia. *Neurosurgery* 19:610-613, 1986.

91. Schultz DR: Occipital neuralgia. *J Am Osteopath Assoc* 76:335-343, 1977.

92. Weed ND: When shoulder pain isn't bursitis. *Postgrad Med* 74:97-104, 1983.

93. Travell JG: Rapid relief of acute "stiff neck" by ethyl chloride spray. *J Am Medical Women's Association* 4:89-95, 1949.

94. Weeks VD, Travell JG: Postural vertigo due to trigger areas in the sternocleidomastoid muscle. *J Pediatr* 47:315-327, 1955.

95. Lewit K: Postisometric relaxation in combination with other methods of muscular facilitation and inhibition. *Manual Medicine* 2:101-104, 1986.

96. Brown BR: Diagnosis and therapy of common myofascial syndromes. *JAMA* 239:646-648, 1978.

97. Lewith GT, Machin D: A randomized trial to evaluate the effect of infra-red stimulation of local trigger points, versus placebo, on the pain caused by cervical osteoarthrosis. *Acupunc Electro-ther Res* 6:277-284, 1981.

98. Waylonis GW: Long-term follow-up on patients with fibrositis treated with acupuncture. *The Ohio State Medical Journal* 73 (May):299-302, 1977.

99. Brown BR: Myofascial and musculoskeletal pain. *Int Anesthesiol Clin* 21:139-151, 1983.

100. Danneskiold-Samsoe B, Christiansen E, Lund B, et al: Regional muscle tension and pain ("fibrositis"): Effect of massage on myoglobin in plasma. *Scan J Rehabil Med* 15:17-20, 1983.

101. Travell JG: Pain mechanisms in connective tissue. In Ragan.C: *Connective Tissues, Transactions of The Second Conference,* May 24-25, 1951. New York, Josiah Macy Jr. Foundation, 1952.

102. Travell JG, Simons, DG: *Myofascial Pain and Dysfunction: The Trigger Point Manual: The Lower Extremities.* vol. 2. Baltimore, MD, Williams & Wilkins, 1992.

103. Manheim CJ, Lavett DK: Chronic Pain as a Reflection of Post-Traumatic Stress Disorder. Proceedings of the World Confederation for Physical Therapy, 11th International Conference. Book II. London, 1991.

104. Barr ML, Kiernan JA: *The Human Nervous System; An Anatomical Viewpoint.* Philadelphia, Harper & Row, Publishers, 1983.

105. Brieg A: *Biomechanics of the CNS: Some Basic Pathological Phenomena.* Stockholm, Alquist & Wiksell, 1960.

106. Brieg A: Biomechanical considerations in the straight leg raising test. *Spine* 4:242-250, 1979.

107. Brieg A, Marions, O: Biomechanics of the lumbosacral nerve roots. *Acta Radiol* 1:1141-1160, 1963.

108. Charnley J: Orthopaedic signs in the diagnosis of disc protrusion with special reference to the straight-leg-raising test. *Lancet* 1:186-192, 1951.

109. Reid J: Ascending nerve roots and tightness of dura. *NZ Med J* 57:16-26, 1958.

110. Frykholm R: Cervical epidural structures, periradicular and epineural sheath. *Acta Chir Scand* 102:10-20, 1951.

111. Cyriax J: *Textbook of Orthopaedic Medicine,* vol 1, 7th ed. London, Balliere Tindall, 1978.

112. Edgar M, Nundy S: Innervation of spinal dura mater. *J Neurol Neurosurg Psychiatry* 29:530-534, 1966.

113. Massey AE: Movement of pain-sensitive structures in the neural canal, in Grieve GP(ed): *Modern Manual Treatment of The Vertebral Column.* London, Churchill Livingston, 1986.

114. Tucker LE: Diagnosis: back pain of extraspinal origin. *Hospital Medicine* April, 1981.

115. Rex LH: Introduction to muscle energy technique. URSA Foundation Course Notes. 1987.

Additional References

Awad EA: Interstitial myofibrositis: Hypothesis of the mechanism. *Arch Phys Med* 54:449-453, 1973.

Baker BA: The Muscle Trigger: Evidence of overload injury. *Journal of Neurology and Orthopaedic Medicine and Surgery* 7:35-43, 1986.

Bartoli V, Dorigo B. Grisillo D, et al: Fibrositic myofascial pain in intermittent claudication: Significance of trigger areas in the calf. *Angiology* 31:11-20, 1980.

Bengtsson A, Henriksson KG, Jorfeldt L, et al: Primary fibromyalgia: A clinical and laboratory study of 55 patients. *Scand J Rheumatol* 29:817-821, 1986.

Bengtsson A, Henriksson KG, Larson J. Muscle biopsy in primary fibromyalgia. *Scand J Rheumatol* 15:1-6, 1986.

Bennet RM: The fibrositis/fibromyalgia syndrome: Current issues and prospectives. *Am J Med* 81(supp 3A):43-49, 1986.

Benoit P, Belt WD: Some effects of local anesthetic agents on skeletal muscle. *Exp Neurol* 34:264-278, 1972.

Bourne IHJ: Treatment of painful conditions of the abdominal wall with local injections. *Practitioner* 224:921-925, 1980.

Brooke RI, Stenn PG: Postinjury myofascial pain dysfunction syndrome: Its etiology and prognosis. *Oral Surgery* 45:846-850, 1978.

Brooke RI, Stenn PG, Mothersill KJ: The diagnosis and conservative treatment of myofascial pain dysfunction syndrome. *Oral Medicine* 44:844-85, 1977.

Brown T, Nemiah JC, et al: Psychologic factors in low-back pain. *N Eng J Med* 251:123-128, 1954.

Bunch RW: Appeal to intelligence and common sense. *Physical Therapy Bulletin* May 11, 1988.

Bunch RW: Myofascial release traced back decades. *Physical Therapy Bulletin* February 17, 1988.

Cheney FD: Muscle tenderness in 100 consecutive psychiatric patients. *Diseases of the Nervous System* 30:478-481, 1969.

Chopra, D: *Ageless Body, Timeless Mind: The Quantum Alternative to Growing Old.* New York, Harmony Books, 1993.

Chopra, D: *Perfect Health: The Complete Mind/Body Guide.* New York, Harmony Books, 1991.

Cohen SR: Follow-up evaluation of 105 patients with myofascial pain-dysfunction syndrome. *J Am Den Assoc* 97:825-828, 1978.

Colton, H: *Touch Therapy.* New York, Kensington Publishing Corp, 1983.

Cooper AL: Trigger-point injection: Its place in physical medicine. *Arch Phys Med Rehabil* 704-709, Oct 1961.

Cooper BC, Alleva M, Cooper DL, et al: Myofascial pain dysfunction: Analysis of 476 patients. *Laryngoscope* 96:1099-1106, 1986.

Crockett DJ, Foreman ME, Alden L, et al: A comparison of treatment modes in the management of myofascial pain dysfunction syndrome. *Biofeedback and Self-Regulation* 11:279-291, 1986.

Cubelli R. Caselli M. Neri M: Pain endurance in unilateral cerebral lesions. *Cortex* 20:369-375, 1984.

Danneskiold-Samsoe B, Christiansen E, Andersen RB: Myofascial pain and the role of myoglobin. *Scand J Rheumatol* 15:154-178, 1986.

De Jong RH: Defining pain terms. *JAMA* 244:143, 1980.

Dorigo B, Bartoli V, Grissillo D, et al: Fibrositic myofascial pain in intermittent claudication. Effect of anesthetic block of trigger points on exercise tolerance. *Pain* 6:183-190, 1979.

Dorko B: Craniosacral therapy and reason. *Physical Therapy Bulletin* 5, March 9, 1988.

Dweck J: Anger blocked by fear. *Energy and Character* 7:32-40, 1980.

Edmond SL: *Manipulation & Mobilization: Extremity and Spinal Techniques.* St. Louis, Mosby, 1993.

Engel, GL: "Psychogenic" pain and the pain-prone patient. *Am J Med* 26:899-918, 1959.

Esposito CJ, Veal SJ, Farman AG: Alleviation of myofascial pain with ultrasonic therapy. *Journal Prosthet Dent* 51:106-108, 1984.

Feldenkrais M: *Awareness Through Movement*. New York, Harper & Row, Publishers, 1977.

Fischer AA: The present status of neuromuscular thermography. *Postgrad Med* special number 79:26-33, 1986.

Fischer AA: Pressure threshold meter: Its use for quantification of tender spots. *Arch Phys Med Rehabil* 67:836-838, 1986.

Fischer AA: Letter to the editor. *Pain* 1987; 28:411-414.

Fordyce WE: A behavioral perspective on chronic pain. *Br J Clin Psychol* 21:313-320, 1982.

Frykholm R: Cervical nerve root compression resulting from disc degeneration and root-sleeve fibrosis. *Act Chir Scand* 160(supp):158-159, 1951.

Gassler JH: If it works, it's for different reasons. *Physical Therapy Bulletin* 3:7, April 27, 1988.

Goddard MD, Reid JD: Movements induced by straight leg raising in the lumbo-sacral roots, nerves and plexus, and in the intrapelvic section of the sciatic nerve. *J Neurol Neurosurg Psychiatry* 28:12-17, 1965.

Graff-Radford SB, Reeves JL, Jaeger B: Management of head and neck pain: Effectiveness of altering factors perpetuating myofascial pain. *Postgrad Med,* 1985; 77:149-158.

Gunn CC: Type IV acupuncture points. *American Journal of Acupuncture* 5:51-52, 1977.

Hallin RP: Sciatic pain and the piriformis muscle. *Postgrad Med,* 1983; 74:69-72.

Hecaen H, Albert M: *Human Neuropsychology*. New York, Wiley, 1978.

Hubbell SL, Thomas M: Postpartum cervical myofascial pain syndrome: Review of Four Patients. *Obstet Gynecol* 65 (supp 3):565-575, 1985.

Hunter C: Myalgia of the abdominal wall. *Can Med Assoc J* 157-161, Feb, 1983.

Ignelzi RJ, Atkinson JH: Pain and its modulation. Part 1. Afferent mechanisms. *Neurosurgery* 6:577-583, 1980.

Ignelzi RJ, Atkinson JH: Pain and its modulation. Part 2. Efferent mechanisms. *Neurosurgery* 6:584-590, 1980.

Kaptchuk, T, Croucher, M: *The Healing Arts: Exploring the Medical Ways of the World*. New York, Summit Books, 1987.

Kellgren JH: Deep pain sensibility. *Lancet* June: 943-949, June 1949.

Kellgren JH: Observations on referrel pain arising from muscle. *Clin Sci* 3:175-190, 1939.

Kelly M: Lumbago and abdominal pain. *Med J Aust* 1:311-317, 1942.

Kepner, JI: *Body Process: Working With the Body in Psychotherapy*. San Francisco, Jossey-Bass Publishers, 1993.

Kraft GH, Johnson EW, LaBan MM: The fibrositis syndrome. *Arch Phys Med Rehabil* 49:155-162, 1968.

Krout RR: Trigger points. *J Am Podiatr Med Assoc* 77:269, 1987.

Laskin DM, Block S: Diagnosis and treatment of myofascial pain-dysfunction (MPD) syndrome. *J Prosthet Dent* 56:75-84, 1986.

Lethem JPD, Salde, JDG, Troup, et al: Outline of a fear-avoidance model of exaggerated pain perception. *Behav Res Ther* 21:401-408, 1983.

Lewit K: The needle effect in the relief of myofascial pain. *Pain* 6:83-90, 1979.

Long C, II: Myofascial pain syndromes. Part I: General characteristics and treatment. *Henry Ford Hosp Med Bulletin* 4:189-192, 1956.

Long C, II: Myofascial pain syndromes. Part II: Syndromes of the head, neck and shoulder girdle. *Henry Ford Hosp Med Bulletin* 3:22-28, 1955.

Mance D, McConnell B, Ryan PA, et al: Myofascial pain syndrome. *J Am Podiatr Med Assoc* 76:328-331, 1986.

Melnick J: Trigger areas and refractory pain in duodenal ulcer. *NY State J Med* 57:1073-1076, 1957.

Melzack R: Myofascial trigger points: Relation to acupuncture and mechanisms of pain. *Arch Phys Med Rehabil* 62:114-117, 1981.

Murray GR, Durh, DCL: Myofibrositis as a simulator of other maladies. *Lancet* 113-116, Jan 1929.

Nel H: Myofascial pain-dysfunction syndrome. *J Prosthet Dent* 40:438-441, 1978.

Perl ER: Sensitization of nociceptors and its relation to sensation. In Bonica JJ, Albe-Fessard D (eds): *Advances in Pain Research and Therapy*. Vol 1. New York, Raven Press, 1976.

Perl ER: Unraveling the story of pain. In Fields, HL (ed): *Advances in Pain Research and Therapy*. Vol 9. New York, Raven Press, 1985.

Price DD, Harkins SW, Baker C: Sensory-affective relationships among different types of clinical and experimental pain. *Pain* 28:297-307, 1987.

Reeves JL, Jaeger B, Graff-Radford SB: Reliability of the pressure algometer as a measure of myofascial trigger point sensitivity. *Pain* 24:313-321, 1986.

Reynolds MD: The development of the concept of fibrositis. *J Hist Med Allied Sci* 38:5-35, 1983.

Reynolds MD: Myofascial trigger point syndromes in the practice of rheumatology. *Arch Phys Med Rehabil* 62:111-114, 1981.

Shpuntoff H: Biofeedback electromyography and inhibition release in myofascial pain dysfunction cases. *NY J Dent* 47:304-309, 1977.

Simons DG: Myofascial trigger points: A need for understanding. *Arch Phys Med Rehabil* 62:97-99, 1981.

Simons DG: Myofascial pain syndromes due to trigger points: 1. Principles, diagnosis and perpetuating factors. *Manual Medicine* 1:67-71, 1985.

Simons DG: Myofascial pain syndromes due to trigger points: 2. Treatment and single-muscle syndromes. *Manual Medicine* 1:72-77, 1985.

Simons DG, Travell JG: Myofascial trigger points: A possible explanation. *Pain* 10:106-109, 1981.

Sjaastad O, Saunte C, Graham JR: Chronic paroxysmal hemicrania. VII. Mechanical precipitation of attacks: New cases and localization of trigger points. *Cephalogia* 4:113-118, 1984.

Sola AE: Treatment of myofascial pain syndromes. In Benedetti C (ed): *Advances in Pain Research and Therapy*. Vol 7. New York, Raven Press, 1984.

Sola AE: Trigger point therapy. In Roberts JR, Hedges JR (eds): *Clinical Procedures in Emergency Medicine*, Philadelphia, WB Saunders, 1985.

Sola AE, Rodenberg ML, Gettys BB: Incidence of hypersensitive areas in posterior shoulder muscles. *Am J Phys Med* 34:585-590, 1955.

Sola AE, Williams RL: Myofascial pain syndromes. *Neurology* 6:91-95, 1956.

Styf J, Lysell E: Chronic compartment syndrome in erector spinae muscle. *Spine* 12:680-682, 1987.

Talaat AM, El-Dibany, MM, El-Garf A: Physical therapy in the management of myofascial pain dysfunction syndrome. *Ann Otol Rhinol Laryngol* 95:225-228, 1986.

Torebjork HE, Ocho, JL, Shady W: Referred pain from intraneural stimulation of muscle fascicles in the median nerve. *Pain* 8:145-156, 1984.

Trager, M, Guadagno, C: Trager Mentastics: *Movement As A Way to Agelessness*. Barrytown, NY, Station Hill Press, Inc, 1987.

Travell JG: Myofascial trigger points: clinical view. In Bonica JJ, Albe-Fessard (ed): *Advances in Pain Research and Therapy*. Vol 1. New York Raven Press, 1976.

Trott PH, Gross AN: Physiotherapy in diagnosis and treatment of myofascial pain dysfunction syndrome. *Int J Oral Surg* 7:360-365, 1978.

Troup JDG, Slade PD: Fear avoidance and chronic musculoskeletal pain. *Stress Medicine* 1:217-220, 1985.

Webber TD: Diagnosis and modification of headache and shoulder-arm-hand syndrome. *J Am Osteopath Assoc* 72:697-710, 1973.

Weinstein G: The diagnosis of trigger points by thermography. *Academy of Neuro-muscular Thermography: Clinical Proceedings, Postgraduate Medicine*. Custom Communications, 1986.

Wolfe F: The clinical syndrome of fibrositis. *Am J Med* 81 (Suppl 3A):7-14, 1986.

Wolfe F, Cathey MA: Prevalence of primary and secondary fibrositis. *J Rheumatol* 10:965-968, 1983.

Wolff BB, Langley S: Cultural factors and the response to pain: A Review. *American Anthropologist* 70:494-501, 1968.

Zohn DA: The quadratus lumborum: An unrecognized source of back pain, clinical and thermographic aspects. *Orthopaedic Review* 15:87-92, 1985.

Suggested Reading

Bass E, Davis L: *The Courage to Heal: A Guide for Women Survivors of Child Sexual Abuse.* New York, Harper & Row Publishers, 1988.

Blume, ES: *Secret Survivors: Uncovering Incest and Its Aftereffects in Women.* New York, John Wiley and Sons, 1990.

Briere JN: *Child Abuse Trauma: Theory and Treatment of the Lasting Effects.* Newbury Park, CA, Sage Publications, Inc, 1992.

Heslin R, Alper T: Touch, A Bonding Gesture. In Wiemann AM, Harrison RP, eds: *Nonverbal Interaction.* Beverly Hills, Sage Publications, 1983.

Lew M: *Victims No Longer: Men Recovering From Incest and Other Sexual Child Abuse.* New York, Nevraumont Publishing Co, 1988.

Patterson ML, Powell JL, Lenihan MG: Touch, compliance, and interpersonal affect. *Journal of Nonverbal Behavior* 10:1:41-50, 1986.

Index

192   The Myofascial Release Manual, Second Edition

Skin Roll, 130
sciatica, 122
scoliosis, 162
serratus anterior, 103
short neck extensors, 62, 68
Simons, 123
Skin Roll, 80, 89, 127
Slump Test, 145
Somato-Emotional Release, 8, 12
spasm, 10, 122
sternocleidomastoid, 61, 69-70, 123
straight leg raising, 146
Strumming, 136-142
subdeltoid bursitis, 122
subclavian artery, 14, 62

temporomandibular joint, 95, 122
TENS, 123, 136
tensor fascia lata, 138
Thoracic Inlet Release, 71-74, 148
Thoracic Inlet Syndrome, 122
tinnitus, 122
torticollis, 122
Travell, 123
triceps, 25
trigger points, 66, 70, 120-123, 138

active, 66, 70, 120-121
definition, 120
effects, 121-123
latent, 121, 123
mimicking symptoms, 121-122
reflex inhibition, 122-123
satellite, 118, 121, 123-124
scar tissue, 122
secondary, 118, 121, 123-124
splinting due to, 121, 124
Trigger Point Release, 5, 61, 66, 122-127, 135, 139, 156, 158
trochanteric bursitis, 122

ultrasound, 123
upper trapezii, 46-49, 103, 107, 109, 111, 113
Upledger, 12

vasoconstriction, 120
vasodilatation, 120
vertebral artery
compression, 16-17
disease, 14, 16
vertigo, 122
vomiting, 122